The Language of Mental Health

This series brings together rich theoretical and empirical discussion at the intersection of mental health and discourse/conversation analysis. Situated broadly within a social constructionist perspective, the books included within this series will offer theoretical and empirical examples highlighting the discursive practices that surround mental health and make 'real' mental health constructs. Drawing upon a variety of discourse and conversation analysis perspectives, as well as data sources, the books will allow scholars and practitioners alike to better understand the role of language in the making of mental health.

We are very grateful to our expert editorial board who continue to provide support for the book series. We are especially appreciative of the feedback that they have provided on earlier drafts of this book. Their supportive comments and ideas to improve the book have been very helpful in our development of the text. They continue to provide support as we continue to edit the book series 'the language of mental health'. We acknowledge them here in alphabetical order by surname.

More information about this series at
http://www.palgrave.com/gp/series/15193

Trini Stickle
Editor

Learning from the Talk of Persons with Dementia

A Practical Guide to Interaction and Interactional Research

palgrave
macmillan

Editor
Trini Stickle
Western Kentucky University
Bowling Green, KY, USA

The Language of Mental Health
ISBN 978-3-030-43976-7 ISBN 978-3-030-43977-4 (eBook)
https://doi.org/10.1007/978-3-030-43977-4

Cover credit: oxygen/gettyimages

This Palgrave Macmillan imprint is published by the registered company Springer Nature Switzerland AG
The registered company address is: Gewerbestrasse 11, 6330 Cham, Switzerland

This book is dedicated to the families and other caregivers who each and every day find ways to alleviate the struggles of and bring moments of joy to persons experiencing dementia.

Acknowledgments

I want to thank all the people who contributed in making this collection possible. As a first time editor, I thank the publishers for supporting the proposal and seeing the potential in this work so quickly. Along with the publishers and their wonderful staff who provided support and guidance, I want to thank the series editors Michelle O'Reilly and Jessica Nina Lester, both of whom have been my steadfast partners in guiding this book from idea to completion. I so very much enjoy our work together on this and our other projects.

Likewise, I have relied on my colleagues' expertise across lands and oceans as I navigated through this inaugural process. For ease, I list them in alphabetical order as they have all been incredibly helpful and for which I thank them:

- Boyd Davis, Bonnie E. Cone Professor of Teaching, English, UNC, Charlotte
- Jacqueline Guendouzi, Department Head, Professor of Communication Sciences and Disorders, Southeastern Louisiana University
- Lisa Mikesell, Associate Professor of Communication, Rutgers

- Nicole Müller, Professor of Speech and Hearing Sciences at University College Cork, Ireland
- Robert W. Schrauf, Department Head of Applied Linguistics, Penn State University
- Anja Wanner, Department Chair of English, University of Wisconsin-Madison
- Alison Wray, Research Professor, School of English, Communication and Philosophy, Cardiff University

I thank also my colleagues at Western Kentucky University for their overwhelming support and excitement not just for my projects but for each member's research and/or creative activities within the Department of English.

Most importantly, I would not be successful without the incredible love and support from my family. My husband, Doug, who not only lives with, and mostly tolerates, the business of this academic life but also makes me be still long enough and often enough to ponder the really important things in our lives, particularly our love and life together. I thank my daughter, son-in-law, and grandchildren who provide an oasis of endless fun and love. And, my son, who with brevity and wit, appreciates my work and reminds me that before all this, I was a good mom.

Contents

Contributors

Boyd H. Davis University of North Carolina, Charlotte, NC, USA

Michael Halpin Department of Sociology and Social Anthropology, Dalhousie University, Halifax, NS, Canada

Heidi E. Hamilton Department of Linguistics, Georgetown University, Washington, DC, USA

Adrienne R. Isaac Department of Linguistics, Georgetown University, Washington, DC, USA

Gunilla Jansson Department of Swedish Language and Multilingualism, Stockholm University, Stockholm, Sweden

Cary J. Kohlenberg Waukesha, USA

Nathaniel J. Kohlenberg Thomas Jefferson University Hospital, Philadelphia, PA, USA

Lyndsay Lindley Department of Social Policy and Social Work, University of York, York, UK

Margaret Maclagan University of Canterbury, Christchurch, New Zealand

Nicole Müller University College Cork, Cork, Ireland; Linköping University, Linköping, Sweden

Charlene Pope Ralph A. Johnson VA Medical Center, Charleston, SC, USA

Norann Richard Clinical Psychologist, CBI Health Centre, Halifax, NS, Canada

Michael Sean Smith Linköping University, Linköping, Sweden

Trini Stickle Western Kentucky University, Bowling Green, KY, USA

Anja Wanner University of Wisconsin-Madison, Madison, WI, USA

Abbreviations

AD	Alzheimer's Disease
ADORE	Alzheimer's and Dementia Outreach, Recruitment, and Engagement Resources
AMTS	Abbreviated Mental Test Score
ARTZ	Artists for Alzheimer's
CA	Conversation Analysis
CAG	Cytosine-Adenine-Guanine
CCC	Carolinas Conversations Collection
DA	Discourse Analysis
DeNDRoN	Dementia and Neurodegenerative Research Network
DLB	Dementia by Lewy Body or Lewy Body Dementia
DSM-III/3	The Diagnostic and Statistical Manual of Mental Disorders, Third Edition
DSM-V/5	The Diagnostic and Statistical Manual of Mental Disorders, Fifth Edition
FTD	Frontotemporal Dementia
HD	Huntington Disease
HIPAA	Health Insurance Portability and Accountability Act (U.S. Congress, 1996)
IRB	Institutional Review Board

LGSWE	Longman Grammar of Spoken and Written English (Biber et al., 1999)
LOAD	Late Onset Alzheimer's disease
MMSE	Mini-Mental State Examination
MoCA	Montreal Cognitive Assessment
NCD	Neurocognitive disorders
NIA	National Institutes of Aging
OED	Oxford English Dictionary
PD	Parkinson's Disease
POGOe	The Portal of Geriatrics Online Education
PWD	Person with Dementia
SLUMS	St. Louis University Mental Status Examination
VA	Veterans Administration (United States)
VaD	Vascular Dementia
WHO	World Health Organization

List of Figures

List of Tables

1
Introduction

Trini Stickle

Aims and Objectives

Learning from the Talk of Persons with Dementia: A Practical Guide to Interaction and Interactional Research aims to provide readers with an understanding of how social-oriented research can bring to light certain conversational practices that may assist clinicians, caregivers, and family members in their interactions with persons with dementia. Our object of study is the conversation between persons with dementia and those with whom they interact. Our goals are to identify, better understand, and share those conversation strategies used by clinicians, caregivers, and family that may prove more conducive than others to building and maintaining relationships with those afflicted by dementia. We might consider, for instance, whether there are certain ways a caregiver can start a conversation that is more likely to elicit a response. In other cases, we observe the value of continuing a conversation despite unexpected and

T. Stickle (✉)
Western Kentucky University, Bowling Green, KY, USA
e-mail: trini.stickle@wku.edu

T. Stickle (ed.), *Learning from the Talk of Persons with Dementia*,
The Language of Mental Health, https://doi.org/10.1007/978-3-030-43977-4_1

occasionally jarring or confusing language from the person with dementia. This interactional approach differs from the clinical and biological types of work with which many may be more familiar. Work such as that on the neurocellular characteristics or potential genetic dispositions of the disease is valuable, indeed crucial, in their own right. But such work can offer little advice on how we might best navigate day-to-day interactions with persons with dementia. We offer this work as part of a continuing effort to provide guidance and hope, if only in some yet small way, to those for whom such conversations have become part of their daily lives.

As the book provides practical guidance to those who interact with persons with dementia, that guidance may take the form of concrete recommendations to specific groups such as caregivers or family members; additionally, it may inform novice researchers who are considering employing any of the methodologies used. Given the potentially wide audience, we have balanced the analyses and sometimes necessary technical terms with pedagogically-oriented sections in each chapter that should prove useful to those coming from backgrounds different from the respective authors. Even if you are not a specialist in some area related to dementia work, rest assured, these sections were written with you also in mind.

Each chapter, for instance, begins with clearly stated learning objectives that largely steer clear of technical jargon. At frequent points throughout the book, you will find various aids to assist your understanding. Some authors use "Thinking Point" boxes to share vignettes and questions for consideration; others use these to summarize and reinforce the chief lessons from the detailed analyses. Some contributors use "Activity" boxes to suggest helpful exercises for use in the classroom, home, and workplace. And, finally, each chapter closes with "Practical Highlights" that summarize the key "take away" messages of that chapter.

Methodological Approaches to Dementia

Before turning to an overview of the individual chapters, I want to first briefly review the methodological approaches you will encounter. The social-interactional research reported here focuses on discourse, or language in use, as the social phenomenon in which meanings are collaboratively made and actions are achieved (see Edwards & Potter, 1992). The term "language in use" may seem unusual, at first. For our purposes, it refers to spoken language used in the "real world" day-to-day. (This stands in contrast to the oftentimes more theoretical study of language conducted by some linguists and philosophers.) Put simply, through our use of language, in conversation with others, we arrive at various understandings of both the larger social world and our conversation partners, and our conversations can allow us to move to other social activities. More specifically, we study the language used in conversation to draw conclusions about the mechanics of language, about how linguistic structures are employed within actual interaction, and to identify how language use helps achieve actions (e.g., accept an invitation, acknowledge a compliment, arrange a meeting).

The methods described below share an emphasis on "language in use." Each, for instance, may combine audio and/or video recordings with detailed transcription of naturally occurring interactions; through this "talk," patterns organically emerge. But the methods oftentimes differ in the way they contextualize the conversation interactions, the importance they place on the environment in which the conversation occurs and the nonlanguage elements of that environment, and in the degree to which they generalize their findings to broader social patterns. Some core elements of those differences follow, but in practice, the methods can overlap significantly.

Discourse Analysis

Discourse analysis (DA) is a close examination of the patterns, themes, and functions of *language in use* as it occurs within particular social contexts. Within the broader social science realm, for instance, discourse analysts might look at how language in use enacts or constructs larger issues of social structure such as identity, power relations, and knowledge. The connection of discourse to social structures and medical or health-related situations has a robust history (e.g., perhaps most notably in Foucault's study of madness, 1972). While some discourse analysts emphasize these broader social issues, others turn greater attention to the ways that language use may function within a conversation beyond its traditional grammatical classifications. In Chapter 5, for example, Davis and Maclagan take this more focused approach and look at how persons with dementia who are exhibiting language impairment can use the words *but* and *so* that a traditional grammarian might simply classify as "conjunctions" and put them to other uses.

Conversation Analysis

Whereas the emphasis in Chapter 5 is on two specific *words* and their use, many of the other contributors in this volume focus on the interconnectedness of participants' *turn of talk* within conversation. They emphasize ways in which one "turn" of talk, with its construction from lexical, syntactic, and prosodic features, engenders another participant's turn—and its unfolding linguistic construction—in the emerging collaborative process of sense making and action. These conversation analytic (CA) methods have been employed profitably in studying, for example, interaction between clinicians and patients (e.g., Goodwin, 2003; Maynard, 2003) and, in the same series as this book, interaction with children with autism (e.g., O'Reilly, Lester, & Muskett, 2016). We find CA methods applied in most of the chapters from Part II.

Ethnography

Ethnography is founded on the principles that social life is meaningful and that social actors create meaning through their interactions, largely, but not exclusively, through language use and the observations of people's behaviors—individually and within group actions. Elements that factor into meaning making are participants' identities, the context of the interaction, and the culture in which the interaction occurs. Data collection traditionally involves observations and subsequent researcher field notes, but technologies such as audio and video recordings are now also used regularly. Some ethnographers also seek insights directly from the participants themselves, employing a series of interviews or collected narratives focused on the research question. Understanding this emic, or insider, perspective allows for another data point from which to look at the relevant issue. This attention to culture and behavior with little or no concern for the turn taking within conversation or the discrete uses of specific words sharply contrasts ethnography from the CA and DA described earlier. However, many of our authors combine elements of the other methods with ethnography. We find an example of the interview approach in Chapter 10, and of ethnography, more generally, in Chapters 7, 8, 9, and 11.

Syntactic Analysis

Syntactic analysis of persons with dementia and other neurocognitive disorders is often conducted on the written, verbal, or computer-mediated responses acquired from the participant through elicitation tasks (see Obler & De Santi, 2000). What is different about the work presented in Chapter 6 is that the syntactic analysis is conducted using a corpus of naturally occurring talk between persons with dementia diagnosis and their unimpaired co-participants. The goal of this analysis is to look at how syntax emerges as a collaborative production in the pursuit of joint actions and how trouble in the syntactic stream of persons with neurocognitive disorders may be facilitated by their co-participants' choice of linguistic resources.

Limitations

The chief limitation one finds here is that case studies of a single or a small collection of similar interactions are common, thus constraining generalizability. Such cases can, however, provide more detailed documentation and refined analysis than large quantitative or experimental studies. Moreover, they can also suggest either a need to develop larger studies or they may be applicable to related problems. Additionally, the nature of our recommendations is such that a clinician or caregiver could, for example, try them with little to no risk. Our goal, then, is not to provide sweeping generalizations but rather nuanced observations that may facilitate better and more frequent interactions with persons suffering from the dementias represented here and also, possibly, from other neurocognitive disorders.

Chapter Overviews

Part I, ***The Talk of Persons with Dementia: What Can It Tell Us?*** consists of chapters two through four and addresses overarching concerns.

Chapter 2: *Dementia, Etiologies, and Implications on Communication* Dementia, a term increasingly being replaced in the medical literature by the phrase "major neurocognitive disorder," affects over 46 million adults worldwide. In this chapter, Kohlenberg and Kohlenberg introduce us to the many causes of dementia, the majority being of the Alzheimer's type, with most other causes attributed to vascular, Lewy body, frontotemporal, or mixed origins. The type and severity of an individual's dementia determine their constellation of symptoms, often categorized as cognitive, functional, and behavioral. There are currently no preventive or curative treatments, and only a handful of pharmacologic options to slow disease progression in those with a progressive etiology. Language has become a diagnostic criterion in the diagnosis of Major Neurocognitive Disorders, per DSM 5, and is now given diagnostic importance equal to that of learning and memory. Communicative deficits may be the harbinger of the illness, or they may occur later in the course, but they will occur. Understanding an individual's type of dementia, with awareness of its natural history, symptom profile, and prognosis is essential. Improving the retained communicative skills of an individual with dementia will increase their quality of life and that of their families or caregivers.

Chapter 3: *Challenges in Collecting Real-World Dementia Discourse* Here Davis and Pope address core questions for researchers to consider when designing and conducting interactional studies of persons with dementia. Topics include the recruiting of research subjects, ethical concerns and issues of consent, and other data collection protocols. While written primarily for the research audience, caregivers and family members may also benefit from this chapter, particularly as they work to elicit and sustain conversations or use talk to better achieve desired actions from persons with dementia.

Chapter 4: ***Why Use Interactional Data to Better Understand the Effects of Dementia?***
Neuropsychological testing is used in the diagnosis and staging of dementia, and it attempts to isolate and measure various aspects of cognitive and linguistic functioning (for instance, working memory, immediate and delayed recall, selective attention, naming, and so forth). Such tests can indeed provide useful staging posts, but they don't tell us much about how persons with (or indeed without) dementia manage to interact and problem solve in their daily lives. Context-embeddedness is a default characteristic of human cognition. People use affordances in their environment to think, learn, remember, and problem solve. Among the tools we use are the physical environment, tools specifically designed to help us remember and problem solve (e.g., shopping lists, calculators), and, most importantly, other people with whom we communicate. Therefore, if we want to find out how well a person functions in daily life, the most useful object of analysis is interaction. This chapter by Müller helps set the scene for the chapters that follow. It outlines a contextualized, interactional perspective on cognition that includes language as a primary cognitive tool, and it formulates strategies and challenges for the investigation of cognition in interaction.

In Part II, ***Learning from the Talk of Persons with Dementia: Practical Steps for Doing and Applying Linguistic and Social Interactional Research***, the focus turns to detailing and discussing actual interactions between persons with dementia and their conversation partners.

Chapter 5: ***Signposts, Guideposts, and Stalls: Pragmatic and Discourse Markers in Dementia Discourse***
As working memory and ability to initiate full conversational gambits begin to decrease, persons with dementia use other features of talk to stay engaged with their conversation partners. Instead of focusing on

content words, which may be either hard to retrieve or to set into an appropriate context, the persons with dementia may exploit pragmatic and discourse markers, the study of which is often neglected by researchers. In this chapter, Davis and Maclagan remedy this neglect with a focus on the pragmatic markers *but* and *so*. In doing so, they illustrate how paying attention to "little words" pays off.

Chapter 6: ***Making Sense of Syntactic Error in Conversations Between Persons with Dementia and Their Non-impaired Co-participants***
In this chapter, Stickle and Wanner demonstrate how syntactic analysis combines with interactional methods to form a tool in understanding the language produced by persons with dementia. Building on earlier findings of syntactic resilience in persons with dementia, they discuss the relationship between syntactic structure and interactional behavior in conversations. Specifically, they present two cases of persons with dementia exhibiting great language impairment symptomatic of late-stage disease. They show that when co-participants respond to impaired syntax as if it made sense, then the participant with dementia may be able to employ better communicative language (if only briefly).

Chapter 7: ***Foregrounding Competence in Interaction with a Person with Dementia: Co-participant Responses to Disordered Talk***
Lindley's chapter highlights how a person's independence may be facilitated, social interaction sustained, and personhood validated during conversations. Through ethnographic observations and close analysis of conversations, Lindley documents everyday practices—alignment, repair, and correction— that can be used by family members to encourage use of both retained interactional abilities and social competencies of a person with dementia. She also offers suggestions on how one could respond in respectful ways should trouble arise in the interaction.

Chapter 8: ***Meaningfulness at the Intersection of Knowledge and Environmental Objects: Investigating Interactions in Art Galleries and Residences Involving Persons with Dementia and Their Carers***
In this chapter, Isaac and Hamilton explore discourse patterns within video-recorded gallery tours for individuals with dementia and their companions to shed light on the way knowledge is transformed as participants focus their joint attention on a small number of paintings. Findings show

that gallery visitors' response types (e.g., describing, evaluating, reasoning, recounting personal experiences) correspond to the level of severity of the condition and are shaped by guides' discursive practices. Building on these gallery observations, they turn their attention to communication centered on objects of joint attention (e.g., family photographs and collectibles) within everyday conversations in assisted living residences. Successful interactions are those that accentuate relative cognitive and discursive strengths of individuals with dementia while deemphasizing weaknesses such as word-finding and episodic memory.

Chapter 9: ***Disagreements in Assessment Sequences with Persons Diagnosed with Frontotemporal Dementia***
Smith reports on an ethnographic study of two individuals with right-predominant frontotemporal dementia. Using an ethnomethodologically informed, CA approach, his study, which will be of particular interest to CA researchers, specifically looks at atypical responses to topics requiring assessments, or value statements. For instance, in normal conversation, the question "Isn't that painting beautiful?" tends to elicit a range of certain expected responses at expected times. Awareness of the possibility for atypical responses and timing (ordering or sequential placement) by persons with dementia can temper the conversation partners' expectations so that they do not allow otherwise unexpected responses, which may fall markedly outside norms, to disrupt conversation and the social relationship.

Chapter 10: ***Dementia and the Life Course: Examining Cognitive Decline in a Slowly Progressing Degenerative Illness***
Halpin and Richard examine dementia across the life course in the context of Huntington disease (HD), a slowly progressing and degenerative illness. Their analysis draws on in-depth interviews—numerous excerpts of which they present—with members of the HD community, sampled across the trajectory of HD, and presents four stages of HD cognitive decline and dementia: (1) the presymptomatic phase, wherein individuals with the HD-gene express concerns about symptom emergence; (2) early cognitive decline, wherein individuals with HD notice initial symptoms (e.g., difficulties with abstract thinking); (3) advanced symptoms, wherein cognitive impairments cause extreme difficulties in

communication; and (4) terminal symptoms, wherein individuals are almost completely unable to communicate. At each stage, the authors provide suggestions for both social science researchers and health professionals working with individuals developing dementia and cognitive impairment. The chapter concludes by reflecting on what HD as a case can tell us more generally about dementia research and care.

Chapter 11: ***Public and Private Spaces in Residential Care for Older People***

Jansson addresses a potential problem arising when residential care centers are designed to more closely replicate a "home" environment in order to alleviate some of the negative effects of institutionalizing the care of persons with dementia: what is a place of residence for one person is a place of work for another. Her methodology draws on conversation analysis combined with ethnographic fieldwork to study the conversations between persons with dementia and their caregivers. The chapter (1) describes how the boundaries between private and public space are negotiated and made relevant in conversation as reflected in the care encounter, and (2) illuminates when the characteristics of a home come in conflict with the formal rules and norms posed by the institution. Her analysis calls for a rethinking of the care home as a "home."

Part III, ***Conclusion: Keeping the Conversation Going***, consists of a final chapter and a glossary. Chapter 12 first summarizes some principles intended to inform our selection of interactional choices as we interact with persons with dementia. The chapter then concludes with a sampling of additional resources for research and collaboration. A glossary follows which does not attempt to be exhaustive but does contain several dozen terms, definitions of which may prove useful to those who are not specialists.

Understanding the Transcription System

Transcriptions of talk employ an agreed upon set of symbols that represent or encode *how* the speakers actually say utterances. These general transcription practices are set forth by Jefferson (2004) and provided below in Table 1.1.

Table 1.1 Jefferson transcription symbols

Symbol	Explanation
(.)	When a full stop symbol is surrounded by round brackets, it shows that a micro pause happened in the conversation
(0.2)	A number inside brackets denotes a timed pause. This is a pause long enough to time and subsequently show in transcription
[ ]	Square brackets denote a point where overlapping speech occurs. This shows the exact point in the turn where the overlap or interruption happened
> <	Arrows surrounding talk like these show that the pace of the speech has speeded up
< >	Arrows in this direction show that the pace of the speech has slowed down
()	When rounded brackets are shown with nothing between them, it shows that the words could not be heard by the analyst
((note here))	Double brackets are used to present a note to the reader; for example, it may show that the speaker nods their head, or shakes their hand, or other non-verbal behavior
Under	If the word or part of a word is underlined, it denotes a raise in volume or emphasis
↑	An upward arrow means there is a rise in intonation
↓	A downward arrow means there is a drop in intonation
→	An arrow like this denotes a particular sentence of interest to the analyst
CAPS	Where capital letters appear, it denotes that something was said loudly
=	The equal sign represents latched speech, a continuation of talk
:::	Colons appear to represent elongated speech, a stretched sound

Source Author

Researchers may also use images, line drawings, or photographs (e.g., Chapter 11) to augment their transcription repertoire using symbols and practices as seen in Table 1.2.

Table 1.2 Transcription practices for images, line drawings, photographs

Symbol	Explanation
* * + + Δ Δ	Gestures and descriptions of embodied actions are delimited between two identical symbols (one symbol per participant) and are synchronized with corresponding stretches of talk
---> --->	The action described continues across subsequent lines until the same symbol is reached
≫	The action described begins before the excerpt's beginning
—≫	The action described continues after the excerpt's end
.....	Action's preparation
----	Action's apex is reached and maintained
,,,,,	Action's retraction
ric	Participant doing the embodied action is identified when (s)he is not the speaker
fig #	The exact moment at which a screen shot has been taken is indicated with a specific symbol showing its position within the turn at talk

References

Edwards, D., & Potter, J. (1992). *Discursive psychology*. London, UK: Sage.

Foucault, M. (1972). *The archaeology of knowledge* (A. M. Sheridan Smith, Trans.). New York, NY: Pantheon.

Goodwin, C. (Ed.). (2003). *Conversation and brain damage*. Oxford, UK: Oxford University Press.

Jefferson, G. (2004). Glossary of transcript symbols with an introduction. *Pragmatics and Beyond New Series, 125,* 13–34.

Maynard, D. W. (2003). *Bad news, good news: Conversational order in everyday talk and clinical settings*. Chicago, IL: University of Chicago Press.

Mondada, L. (2014). *Conventions for multimodal transcription*. Retrieved from https://franz.unibas.ch/fileadmin/franz/user_upload/redaktion/Mondada_conv_multimodality.pdf.

Obler, L. K., & De Santi, S. (2000). Eliciting language from patients with Alzheimer's disease. In L. Menn & N. R. Bernstein (Eds.), *Methods for studying language production* (pp. 403–416). Mahwah, NJ: Lawrence Erlbaum and Associates.

O'Reilly, M., Lester, J. N., & Muskett, T. (2016). *Discourse/conversation analysis and autism spectrum disorder*. London, UK: Palgrave.

Part I

The Talk of Persons with Dementia: What Can It Tell Us?

2

Dementia, Etiologies, and Implications on Communication

Cary J. Kohlenberg and Nathaniel J. Kohlenberg

Learning Objectives

By the end of this chapter, you will be able to:

- Better understand and identify different dementias, their symptoms, and causes;
- Appreciate the neurological and social changes that persons with dementia may be experiencing.

C. J. Kohlenberg (✉)
Waukesha, USA
e-mail: cjkohlenberg@ipcResearch.org

N. J. Kohlenberg
Thomas Jefferson University Hospital, Philadelphia, PA, USA
e-mail: nxk089@jefferson.edu

T. Stickle (ed.), *Learning from the Talk of Persons with Dementia*,
The Language of Mental Health, https://doi.org/10.1007/978-3-030-43977-4_2

Thinking Points: Vignette 1

- Clara has been exhibiting gradual, progressive word finding difficulties and general forgetfulness for over three years. Her late husband wasn't troubled by this. Instead, during this time, he simply had taken over most of the driving, household chores, and financial management. Still, these accommodations changed their relationship, and those changes occasionally led to Clara feeling more of a dependent, child-like, than a partner.
  Question: What may be causing these changes seen in Clara?
- After their father's death one year ago, Clara's children now had the opportunity to notice these behaviors in their mother. They assumed that these changes along with increased anxiety and seemingly "initial" bouts of confusion were due to grief. They were not aware of how long their mother had been experiencing these symptoms or the many responsibilities that their father had assumed due to Clara's increasing difficulties negotiating the world around her.
  Question: What else may Clara's children have been missing?
- The children watched as Clara's conversations were increasingly challenging—for her and them—as her difficulties expressing herself led to frustration and irritability. They became increasingly concerned when their mother confused their names with her siblings' names, did not acknowledge special days, like their birthdays, and failed to pay her bills. One child stepped in to help manage finances; another visited with her every few days. The children's relationship with their mother was changing. When she got lost while driving, one finally uttered the word and voiced their fear: ***dementia***.
  Question: How should the family best intervene on Clara's behalf?

Introduction

Geriatric psychiatrists routinely treat the cognitive, emotional, functional, and interactional effects of dementia as depicted in Clara's story and the consequence of those changes in the relationships between patients, their families, and the community. From our clinical experience and current research, we focus this chapter on how various neurocognitive disorders (NCD)—their symptoms and progression—affect the interactional abilities of people with dementia and their relationships. We also provide a clinical review of the common forms of dementia with their neurocognitive effects and symptoms. For a complete listing of stages and symptoms, see *The Diagnostic and Statistical Manual of Mental Disorders*, 5th ed. (American Psychiatric Association, 2013). Specifically, this chapter will compare and contrast common dementias and their effects on communication. We will reflect on how such clinical observations can help researchers, various practitioners, care-giving staff, as well as family members, in order that they may better serve people experiencing dementia.

Some Preliminaries: Clinical Description of Dementia

Our understanding and recognition of defining characteristics of dementia continue to evolve. Previous editions of *The Diagnostic and Statistical Manual of Mental Disorders* (DSM III and IV) identified the condition "Dementia" primarily as a group of disorders in which the cardinal symptom was a deficit in short term memory (American Psychiatric Association, 1980, 1994). Now, however, the conditions relating to "dementia or dementias" refer to the conglomerate of symptoms involving one or more cognitive domains and are grouped under the label Major Neurocognitive Disorders (American Psychiatric Association, 2013). Domains affected go beyond memory to include language, executive function, complex attention, perceptual-motor, and social cognition. Per the *DSM 5* definitions, these deficits, whatever the etiology, must be acquired and demonstrate significant decline from a previous level of performance severe enough to interfere with independence in everyday activities. Different etiologies of dementia (Alzheimer's, Lewy body, frontotemporal, and vascular) have additional criteria to differentiate them. Additionally, each type of neurocognitive disorder is classified by severity: Mild or Major. Major severity is further divided into stages of mild, moderate, or severe. Each is distinguished further by the presence or absence of behavioral symptoms. The import of this change is that "dementia" is now categorized as a broader based collection of disorders, all with particular, albeit sometimes overlapping, deficits and declines in functional impairments.

A Brief Look at Common Dementia Etiologies

The most common forms of NCD/dementia include Alzheimer's disease (AD), Lewy body dementia (DLB), frontotemporal dementia (FTD), and vascular dementia (VaD) (Kaufman, Geyer, & Milstein, 2016). The first three are neurodegenerative processes that result from the progressive loss of nerve cells in the brain. VaD may be a sole cause of dementia, but it often co-exists with another neurodegenerative type. Many less frequent causes, such as Huntington's disease (see also Chapter 10), Parkinson's disease, alcohol-related or other injuries, account for the remainder. Additionally, dementia-like symptoms may arise from reversible causes (e.g., infection, pharmacological interactions). While a definitive identification of a dementia cause for a given patient is sought, for better understanding, treatment, and planning, it is not always achievable. Confounding factors include symptom overlap and limitations in our gradually developing brain scan and genetic testing technology.

Diagnostic Procedures

When any form of dementia is suspected, a thorough diagnostic evaluation is mandated. Age of onset, family history, and underlying medical history and risk factors are strong diagnostic indicators. Full evaluation includes physical and neurological examinations, laboratory studies, brain scans, and often neuropsychological testing to evaluate potentially reversible causes of cognitive decline (Chen et al., 2016). (The use of biomarkers is still primarily in research stages, not readily available for clinical evaluation.) Evaluation of reversible dementia typically includes testing for vitamin B12 deficiency, thyroid abnormalities, infection, and assessment of medication side effects or interactions. Psychiatric diagnoses, particularly Major Depression or other Mood Disorders must also be ruled out, as they may present as a primary neurocognitive disorder. Normal aging and senescence are often ruled out as neither impairs communication (Bayles, 1982).

Key, then, to diagnosing dementia is the marked and increasing communication impairments. Most important to this chapter's as well as the text's focus is the semantic system's vulnerability to the effects of a particular progressive dementia. While language abilities of persons with dementia are resilient, particularly the phonological (sounds) and syntactic (grammar) systems, losses in their semantic, pragmatic, and lexical retrieval systems progressively affect their ability to effectively communicate (Murdoch, Chenery, Wilks, & Boyle, 1987).

Thinking Points: Vignette 2

- In addition to Clara's progressive short term memory impairments and loss of independent functioning, she experienced further decline in her communicative abilities. Her sentences have become very simple; she often searches for the next word, often skipping it or using a generic word like "thing" or "it"; and she sometimes misuses pronouns, calling her daughter "he" or her brother "she". Fortunately, her family is still able to understand most of what she is attempting to communicate. **Questions**: How would you as a family member adjust your conversations with Clara? How would you as a clinician advise Clara's family?
- One-on-one interactions are often easier than group conversations. Addressing one topic at a time, being more agreeable and not overly correcting errors and misstatements is suggested (see Chapters 5, 6, 7, and 11).
- Conversations are often helped by being briefer and more focused, particularly as dementia progresses (see Chapters 8, 9, and 10).

A Closer Look at the Individual Etiologies of Dementia

Alzheimer's Disease

AD accounts for 60–80% of all dementias, globally, either as a singular etiology or concomitantly with cerebrovascular disease (Alzheimer's Association, 2018). It is chronic and progressive and ultimately fatal. No preventive, curative, or disease modifying treatments exist. As reported in *2019 Alzheimer's Disease Facts and Figures,* one in ten Americans aged 65 or older has AD, with a total of 5.8 million Americans currently affected (Gaugler, James, Johnson, Marin, & Weuve, 2019). Gaugler and colleagues project that, in the U.S. alone, the prevalence is expected to reach 14 million by 2050 (2019). Worldwide, over 46 million people have dementia (Wang et al., 2016), significantly increased from 36 million (Batsch & Mittelman, 2012). The number is expected to reach 75 million people worldwide by 2030 (Prince et al., 2015).

Neurocognitive Causes and Changes

AD was first identified over 100 years ago by its pathognomonic findings at autopsy of neurofibrillary tangles and neuritic plaques. The tangles are composed of hyperphosphorylated tau and the plaques are made of beta-amyloid. Recent advances have led to a biomarker categorization system, A/T/N, (amyloid/tau/non-specific) based on measures of brain beta-amyloid deposits, phosphorylated tau found in cerebrospinal fluid, and other nonspecific biomarkers of neurodegeneration per brain imaging (Jack et al., 2016). AD neurodegenerative biomarkers are associated with decreased cognitive function but not beta-amyloid in cognitively normal older individuals (Wirth et al., 2013). These have been incorporated into the National Institutes of Aging (NIA) staging guidelines (Sperling et al., 2011) but have yet to become useful in daily practice. A literature into the genetics of AD is emerging, and while a full review is beyond the scope of this chapter, we will briefly summarize.

The only gene identified with Late Onset Alzheimer's Disease (LOAD), defined as onset after age 60, is apolipoprotein E (APOE). APOE is considered a "risk factor" gene because inheriting a certain allele may increase or decrease a person's risk of developing AD: APOE-2 appears to be protective; APOE-3 is the most common allele and appears to be neutral; APOE-4 appears to increase the risk for developing LOAD. Still, the presence or absence of APOE 2, 3, or 4 will not definitively cause or prevent AD (see Shivani, 2015).

Demographic Factors

Age is the key predictive factor: the older persons are, the higher their risk for developing AD becomes. As noted in the 2019 Alzheimer's Disease Facts and Figures report, 3% of people age 65–74, 17% of people age 75–84, and 32% of people age 85 and older have AD; with women experiencing the highest incidence; among people age 71 and older, 16% of women have AD or other dementias compared with 11% of men (Gaugler et al., 2019). African Americans and Hispanics have a higher incidence than Caucasians or Asians with incidence rates for African Americans about twice as likely and Hispanics about 1.5 times as likely as non-Hispanic Whites (Gaugler et al., 2019).

Prognostic Information

AD is viewed as a three-stage continuum (Gaugler et al., 2019). The preclinical stage is defined as having the presence of brain changes, per imaging, without clinical symptoms. Mild Cognitive Impairment (MCI) due to AD is characterized by both brain changes and mild cognitive symptoms that do not significantly affect everyday living. Dementia due to AD presents as brain changes and significant problems with memory, thinking and/or behavior which interfere with daily activities.

AD Symptoms

AD involves progressive short-term memory decline, particularly impacting executive functioning, language, and visuospatial abilities. Anomia, or word finding difficulties, is a frequent early symptom. A decrease in spontaneous verbal output manifests early and worsens as the dementia progresses. Likewise, paraphasic errors (the use of incorrect words or syllables) and certain symptoms of aphasia, such as circumventing forgotten words, are exhibited. Mild AD causes mild word finding problems, word substitution, repetition, and reluctance to speak, generated from fear of mistakes, Moderate AD shows midrange symptoms, with increased repetition, disorganization, gaps in speech, and confabulation. Severe AD causes significant difficulties to be understood, reduced speech often resulting in mutism (for a review, see Kindell, Keady, Sage, & Wilkinson, 2017).

Synchronic memory and neurocognitive decline occur with increasing impairments in functional abilities and behavioral/neuropsychiatric symptoms. Correlating with memory and communication declines, behavioral changes are common, often social withdrawal, apathy, depression and irritability early in the course, with aggression and psychosis in later stages of the disease (Jost & Grossberg, 1996).

Thinking Points: Vignette 3

- Clara's family moved her to a memory care facility. The transition was made easier by incorporating a number of family photos and Clara's personal items. Her children allowed her to talk and repeat herself without interruption. She rarely shows awareness of her deficits.

  Question: How could you as a family member maximize Clara's communication?

  Question: How could you as a clinician guide Clara's family on further expected communicative declines?
- Use of smiles, gestures, and other nonverbals can greatly aid communication. Gently assisting a person who is struggling to find a word is often helpful. However, taking over the conversation can be met with increased frustration and anger. Accept repetition. Allow the person with dementia to lead the conversation with your appropriate guidance. See Chapters 6 and 11.

Lewy Body Dementia

DLB, sometimes referred to as Dementia with Lewy Bodies (DLB), is more frequently recognized, and, due to post-mortem exams, speculated as the most common progressive dementia (Outeiro et al., 2019). While DLB may present as the single cause, it often co-occurs with other dementias. Disambiguating single versus mixed dementia is near impossible as DLB's symptoms overlap with AD and Parkinson's disease. These include memory impairment plus the classic triad of early presentation of prominent visual hallucinations, Parkinsonian symptoms, and fluctuating levels of consciousness or confusion.

DLB Causes

Rather than the plaques and tangles seen in AD, the microscopic findings in DLB are "Lewy bodies" or accumulations of alpha-synuclein, a presynaptic neuronal protein (Stefanis, 2012). These structures are also found in the brains of persons with Parkinson's disease (PD), where their density and locations result in identifiable types and severities of symptoms. For instance, in the basal ganglia, they cause classic PD motor symptoms; in the cortex, they are responsible for memory impairment. Distinguishing DLB from AD is a clinical diagnosis, without any specific findings on laboratory testing or scans. Neuropsychological testing may be helpful for diagnostic clarity.

Language Effects of DLB

As with AD, language related symptoms are not seen in early DLB (Gatchel et al., 2015, p. 191; Muangpaisin, 2007), but other symptoms are key to DLB.

Thinking Points: Vignette 4

- Ruth is a healthy 76-year-old widow, living independently in a senior apartment complex, with no obvious impairments. Her son became concerned when Ruth began talking about the friendly children who visit her in the evening and at night. He knew no children lived in the building, and immediately was skeptical about Ruth's reports. She was not bothered by "the children" and, in fact, looked forward to their "visits."

Question: What course of action should Ruth's son pursue in thinking his mother's reports are delusions?

Question: What causes could delusions be a symptom of?

Egosyntonic (pleasant) visual hallucinations, commonly of children or animals, are often early symptoms of DLB. (In most other forms of dementia, hallucinations do not occur until late stages.) In DLB, people present to their doctor with visual hallucinations or tremors, often before the presence of memory impairment is noted. Prescribing an acetylcholinesterase inhibitor may assist, a person with DLB to live a fairly independent lifestyle long before moving to an assisted living facility.

Frontotemporal Dementias

FTDs are a large group of somewhat similar dementias that affect various parts of the frontal (primarily) and temporal lobes of the brain. While majority of people with AD are over 65 years of age, most people who develop FTDs do so before age 65 with the average onset at 53 years old (Gatchel et al., 2015). Not only do FTDs typically occur earlier in life than AD, but also progression to death is shorter.

FTDs Cause and Predispositions

FTDs often cluster in families (Autosomal Dominant pattern) with up to one half of people having an affected family member. Recent studies have subdivided types of FTDs based on types of proteins found at particular neuro-locations, with symptoms and extent of neurodegeneration mapping to locations (Gatchel et al., 2015).

FTDs Behavioral Effects

The frontal lobes of the brain function as the control centers for personality, emotions, and executive decisions (Kaufman et al., 2016, p. 123). They also work to inhibit socially inappropriate and impulsive behaviors. Thus, advancing FTDs result in changes often characterized as the coarsening of personality, loss of inhibitions, increasing emotionality and problems with organizing, planning, sequencing, and other executive functions. Clinically, people with FTD may have cognitive symptoms similar to those seen in AD, but with much more prominent and early behavioral symptoms, including disinhibition and impulsivity, along with language deficits (see Chapter 9).

Language Effects of FTDs

In contrast to AD, people with FTDs often exhibit early and progressive paraphasias, anomias, and decreased fluency. When the left hemisphere is heavily affected, language symptoms are primary, and manifest significantly earlier than cognitive symptoms (Gatchel et al., 2015, p. 193). Semantic Dementias (also known as Semantic Variant Primary Progressive Aphasia) are types of FTDs highly affecting the left temporal lobe. People with FTDs lose the ability to match certain words with their images or meanings—verbal and nonverbal—but often retain intact fluency and episodic memory (Bayles, 1982).

Thinking Points: Vignette 5

- Tom is a 62-year-old retired engineer. His wife reports that he was always an active, energetic, "type A" person. About 3 years ago, he began exhibiting increasing irritability with his family. He began having trouble "finding the right word" and with concise expression. For the first time in his career, he was reprimanded for making significant mistakes in his work and for treating colleagues in an angry manner. He was not forgetful, and his family first assumed that he must be experiencing depression. He was prescribed an antidepressant medication.
- Tom did not respond to the antidepressant. His irritability worsened. His word finding problems increased and he began making out-of-character, insensitive, and inappropriate comments in public situations. He had more problems with work performance and lost his job. His primary care doctor's evaluation, including blood work and a brain scan, showed no obvious problems.
- Due to Tom's family's insistence, he underwent neuropsychological testing, which yielded a diagnosis of FTD.
  Question: What conditions other than depression might account for Tom's changing behaviors?
- Self and family advocacy in exploring alternative diagnoses and treatment options can be key to accurate identification.

Vascular Dementia

VaD differ from the previously described dementias. VaD was formerly referred to as Multi-Infarct Dementia (MID). VaD's classic progression includes a step-wise decline in cognitive functioning, along with weakness and physical impairments due to a series of strokes. The causes of VaD can range from one large, usually unilateral Cerebrovascular Accident (CVA), to many small strokes occurring over time. Physical deficits such as single-sided paralysis often result. Numerous small strokes, however, may falsely present as a progressive neurodegenerative dementia, as no significant neurological deficits may be obvious without a thorough neurological evaluation. The location, number, and severity of each stroke determine the overall symptom profile including cognitive loss, functional and behavioral symptoms, and language effects. VaD may occur as the single cause of dementia or may co-exist with another neurodegenerative dementia.

VaD Causes and Predisposition

Population based studies document vascular pathologies in 50% of older persons that, consequentially, correlate with other dementia (Kapasi & Schneider, 2016). Genetics can be direct causative factors in VaD, specifically Cerebral Autosomal Dominant Arteriopathy with Subcortical Infarcts and Leukoencephalopathy (CADASIL). However, the most common cause of VaD is stroke, either single or multiple, due to primarily preventable causes: high blood pressure, obesity, elevated cholesterol, and poorly controlled diabetes mellitus.

VaD Prevention

Aggressive management of cardiovascular risk factors such as blood pressure, cholesterol, and blood sugar along with diet and exercise, avoidance of smoking, and minimal alcohol consumption are the most effective preventions. Anticoagulation or antiplatelet treatment may either be recommended or contraindicated per stroke type.

Language Effects of VaD

When vascular damage is predominantly in the left hemisphere, language impairment is typically exhibited, whereas predominantly right sided lesions result in visuospatial problems (Kaufman et al., 2016, p. 155).[1] Location, size, and neurodegenerative comorbidity determine symptom presentation (Gatchel et al., 2015, p. 195).

Thinking Points: Vignette 6

- William is an obese 73-year-old who had smoked two packs of cigarettes daily, and drank alcohol excessively for 40 years. Following a small heart attack at 59 years old, he stopped all cigarette and alcohol use. However, he has slowly gained weight and does not pay attention to his blood sugar or blood pressure. He is increasingly sedentary and just doesn't like to "take pills". His memory and abilities to manage his own finances appear normal. Unfortunately, William has also had a series of strokes. They caused paralysis on one side of his body and significant expressive speech impairments. He appears able to understand other's speech, but communicates best, though not consistently, with gestures, yes/no utterances and pointing to a communication board.

  Question: How do Williams's receptive and expressive communication problems compare with Clara's?

  Question: At this point, would you recommend any specific treatments or interventions?

For degenerative dementias (e.g., Clara's AD, Ruth's DLB), medications (e.g., acetylcholinesterase inhibitors, memantine) can slow progression of communicative, memory, and functional decline. For abrupt and rapid changes caused primarily by VaD, such as William's, these treatments are of no benefit. As highlighted by the many vignettes, cognitive impairment and declines in language ability are the cardinal symptoms of dementia, but physical, behavioral, emotional, and functional impairments likely accompany. Verbal communication with a person with dementia, particularly seen in William's case, can often be enhanced with non-verbal approaches, including gestures, and visual cues and prompts.

[1]The dominant hemisphere controls most language, though the nondominant hemisphere controls prosody, including inflection, rhythm and manner of speaking. The dominant hemisphere also contains the main areas for cognitive activity and emotions (Kaufman et al., 2016, p. 155).

Discussion

No cures for any form of dementia exist. Treatments may result in modest neurocognitive (including language), functional, and/or behavioral improvements, but a more realistic expectation may be a temporary period of stability, followed by a temporary slowing of anticipated decline. (Exceptions are an isolated vascular event, followed by excellent control of future risk factors, or identification of another reversible dementia cause.) Behavioral strategies, especially the setting of regular routines, in simplified familiar environments are highly important. Cognitively stimulating activities are often well accepted by patients and their families, have no adverse effects, and may provide modest help.

What can be done, by those of us who interact with persons experiencing any of these dementias, is to work toward better communication practices. The vignettes provided in this chapter aim to help with that understanding for all stakeholders—fellow practitioners, researchers, caregivers, family members, and the persons struggling with the diseases themselves. These are summarized in the box below.

Practical Highlights

1. Make no assumptions about an individual's cognitive and communicative abilities. But, be acutely aware of progressive declines in a person's memory AND communicative abilities.
2. Reports of "unreal" visualizations can be a warning sign of early DLB or a late sign of other dementias.
3. Drastic changes in personality, particularly lack of inhibition, can be signs of an FTD.
4. Some progressive dementias respond to medications (e.g., AD, DLB) or behavioral changes (e.g., VaD).
5. Advocacy—self or family—is the best assurance for diagnosis and treatment.

Continuing that goal, the research findings that follow in this book aim to provide a window into current interactional and communication strategies beneficial to all who are experiencing the epidemic of dementias: individuals, families, communities—local and global.

References

Alzheimer's Association. (2018). 2018 Alzheimer's disease facts and figures. *Alzheimer's & Dementia, 14*(3), 367–429.

American Psychiatric Association. (1980). *Diagnostic and statistical manual of mental disorders: DSM-III* (3rd ed.). Arlington, VA: American Psychiatric Publishing.

American Psychiatric Association. (1994). *Diagnostic and statistical manual of mental disorders: DSM-IV* (4th ed.). Arlington, VA: American Psychiatric Publishing.

American Psychiatric Association. (2013). *Diagnostic and statistical manual of mental disorders: DSM-5*™ (5th ed.). Arlington, VA: American Psychiatric Publishing.

Batsch, N. L., & Mittelman, M. S. (2012). *World Alzheimer report 2012: Overcoming the stigma of dementia*. London, UK: Alzheimer's Disease International (ADI). Retrieved from https://www.alz.co.uk/research/world-report-2012.

Bayles, K. A. (1982). Language function in senile dementia. *Brain and Language, 16*(2), 265–280.

Chen, G., Shu, H., Chen, G., Ward, B. D., Antuono, P. G., Zhang, Z., & Li, S. J. (2016). Staging Alzheimer's disease risk by sequencing brain function and structure, cerebrospinal fluid, and cognition biomarkers. *Journal of Alzheimer's Disease, 54*(3), 983–993.

Gatchel, J. R., Wright, C. I., Falk, W. E., & Trinh, N. (2015). Dementia. Chapter 19. In T. A. Stern, M. Fava, T. E. Wilens, & J. F. Rosenbaum (Eds.), *Massachusetts general hospital psychopharmacology and neurotherapeutics e-book* (pp. 184–197). London: Elsevier Health Sciences.

Gaugler, J., James, B., Johnson, T., Marin, A., & Weuve, J. (2019). 2019 Alzheimer's disease facts and figures. *Alzheimers & Dementia, 15*(3), 321–387.

Jack, C. R., Bennett, D. A., Blennow, K., Carrillo, M. C., Feldman, H. H., Frisoni, G. B., … Petersen, R. C. (2016). A/T/N: An unbiased descriptive classification scheme for Alzheimer disease biomarkers. *Neurology, 87*(5), 539–547.

Jost, B. C., & Grossberg, G. T. (1996). The evolution of psychiatric symptoms in Alzheimer's disease: A natural history study. *Journal of the American Geriatrics Society, 44*(9), 1078–1081.

Kapasi, A., & Schneider, J. A. (2016). Vascular contributions to cognitive impairment, clinical Alzheimer's disease, and dementia in older persons. *Biochimica et Biophysica Acta (BBA)-Molecular Basis of Disease, 1862*(5), 878–886.

Kaufman, D. M., Geyer, H. L., & Milstein, M. J. (2016). *Kaufman's clinical neurology for psychiatrists E-book* (E-reader version). London: Elsevier Health Sciences.

Kindell, J., Keady, J., Sage, K., & Wilkinson, R. (2017). Everyday conversation in dementia: A review of the literature to inform research and practice. *International Journal of Language & Communication Disorders, 52*(4), 392–406.

Muangpaisin, W. (2007). Clinical differences among four common dementia syndromes. *Geriatrics and Aging, 10,* 425–429.

Murdoch, B. E., Chenery, H. J., Wilks, V., & Boyle, R. S. (1987). Language disorders in dementia of the Alzheimer type. *Brain and Language, 31*(1), 122–137.

Outeiro, T. F., Koss, D. J., Erskine, D., Walker, L., Kurzawa-Akanbi, M., Burn, D., … McKeith, I. (2019). Dementia with Lewy bodies: An update and outlook. *Molecular Neurodegeneration, 14*(1), 5. https://doi.org/10.1186/s13024-019-0306-8.

Prince, M., Wimo, A., Guerchet, M., Ali, G., Wu, Y., Prina, M. (2015). *World Alzheimer report 2015: The global impact of dementia: An analysis of prevalence, incidence, cost and trends.* Retrieved from https://www.alz.co.uk/research/WorldAlzheimerReport2015.pdf.

Shivani, G. (2015). Alzheimer disease and APOE-4. *Medscape.* Retrieved from https://emedicine.medscape.com/article/1787482-overview.

Sperling, R. A., Aisen, P. S., Beckett, L. A., Bennett, D. A., Craft, S., Fagan, A. M., … Park, D. C. (2011). Toward defining the preclinical stages of Alzheimer's disease: Recommendations from the National Institute on Aging-Alzheimer's Association workgroups on diagnostic guidelines for Alzheimer's disease. *Alzheimer's & Dementia, 7*(3), 280–292.

Stefanis, L. (2012). α-synuclein in Parkinson's disease. *Cold Spring Harbor Perspectives in Medicine, 2*(2). Retrieved from http://perspectivesinmedicine.cshlp.org/content/2/2/a009399.full.pdf.

Wang, H., Naghavi, M., Allen, C., Barber, R. M., Bhutta, Z. A., Carter, A., … Coggeshall, M. (2016). Global, regional, and national life expectancy, all-cause mortality, and cause-specific mortality for 249 causes of death, 1980–2015: A systematic analysis for the Global Burden of Disease Study 2015. *The Lancet, 388*(10053), 1459–1544. https://doi.org/10.1016/S0140-6736(16)31012-1.

Wirth, M., Madison, C. M., Rabinovici, G. D., Oh, H., Landau, S. M., & Jagust, W. J. (2013). Alzheimer's disease neurodegenerative biomarkers are associated with decreased cognitive function but not β-amyloid in cognitively normal older individuals. *Journal of Neuroscience, 33*(13), 5553–5563.

3

Challenges in Collecting Real-World Dementia Discourse

Boyd H. Davis and Charlene Pope

Learning Objectives

By the end of this chapter, you will be able to:

- Better plan a research agenda—the question(s) you wish to probe and the strategies for data collection to best accomplish your goals;
- Understand purposes and data collection methods used to achieve research findings;
- Expand ways to elicit discourse, consult research for help, and participate in research protocols.

B. H. Davis (✉)
University of North Carolina, Charlotte, NC, USA
e-mail: bdavis@uncc.edu

C. Pope
Ralph A. Johnson VA Medical Center, Charleston, SC, USA
e-mail: Charlene.Pope@va.gov

T. Stickle (ed.), *Learning from the Talk of Persons with Dementia*,
The Language of Mental Health, https://doi.org/10.1007/978-3-030-43977-4_3

Introduction

Multiple questions arise for researchers wishing to learn from the talk of persons who have dementia diagnoses. The initial challenge in collecting dementia discourse comes from two questions, "Why?" and "How?" Thinking through these questions will help address your purposes and identify the best mode for collecting data. While written primarily for the research audience, caregivers and family members may also benefit from this chapter, particularly as they work to elicit and sustain conversations or use talk to better achieve desired actions from persons with dementia. (Editor's note: People who are not researchers might want particularly to read the section titled "Purposes", especially under the subheadings *Conversation*, *Reminiscence*, and *Activities*.)

As researchers, teachers, and family members of persons with dementia, we have found every purpose for language research with persons with dementia includes multiple facets. Perhaps you want to investigate how people with dementia converse with family members or friends as opposed to how they might talk differently to caregiving staff or medical personnel. Your goal might be to stimulate memories of the past by reminiscing in various formats, perhaps with physical or technological support. Do you hope to design or sponsor special activities, such as visits to museums or the theatre? Are you engaged in medical trials which use discourse to elicit tests of memory, physical ability, or task performance? These are the "*why*" questions. Below, we address "*how*" to help you collect discourse. Next, in the section "Purposes", we briefly discuss examples of how we and other researchers approach collecting discourse for various purposes. The section "Collection Protocols", identifies factors we consider prior to collecting discourse data.

Purposes

This section highlights and summarizes numerous projects and their purposes. For each example, consider the following questions to help you develop a comprehensive research strategy. Each will be further discussed in the section "Collection Protocols":

Thinking Points: Preliminary Questions for Researchers

1. Questions About Recruitment
   (a) How will you locate persons with dementia for research?
   (b) As stigma toward persons with dementia continues to exist, many families do not want others to know that someone in their family has dementia; in addition, many people may feel antipathy toward persons with dementia (Rosato, Levey, Cooper, De Cock, & Devine, 2019). How will you address these issues as you approach prospective volunteers?
   (c) Do you plan to ask persons living in various residential settings, such as assisted living, nursing homes, or memory care units? You will need to obtain consent—possibly at corporate level—to enter their facilities and talk with their residents, and they will expect you to protect the privacy of staff and residents. Acquiring consent is required for community members obtained from support groups (in-person and online), church groups, or persons you may already know (see additional information on consent).
   (d) Would using an existing database of persons with dementia, caregivers, or media text addressing dementia be a good source (e.g., Carolina Conversation Collection: http://carolinaconversations.musc.edu)? (Note: Consent may be needed to use such databases).
   (e) Will you need to verify that persons have a specific condition of dementia and/or the severity of their condition? Such information is not often readily available. You will need to consult the appropriate Internal Review Board (IRB) (e.g., universities) or Board of Ethics (e.g., hospitals) in order to comply with research ethics and the Health Insurance Portability and Accountability Act of 1996 (HIPAA).
2. Ethical Questions and Consent
   (a) How will you protect the rights of your prospective participants and ensure you are abiding by ethical research protocols? Persons with dementia are members of a vulnerable population, and they and their family members must have personal information as well as their personhood protected in order to avoid human rights violations. For example, recommendations have been provided to negotiate informed consent in acute care settings (Holden et al., 2018) and in research on cognitively impaired adults with multiple medical conditions (Prusaczyk, Cherney, Carpenter, & DuBois, 2017).
   (b) Do you know the ethical and legal processes for creating protocols for gaining legal consent or assent from a participant and their guardian? The IRB and the Board of Ethics as well as residence administrators (e.g., nursing homes) can inform you. See also the **ADORE** toolkit website listed in the Recommended Reading section.

3. Equipment
   (a) How will you collect the discourse data? Will you use digital audio- or video-recorders?
   (b) You must establish a process for assuring the security of devices as well as the maintenance of the data you hope to collect. Consult your IRB or Board of Ethics to ensure approval of your process.

Conversation—unscripted, unprompted, spontaneous talk in natural settings—is not always easy to carry on with persons with dementia. "Extreme reactions" (Wray, 2016, p. 116) can come from participants or caregivers, who may not understand the impact of dementia on a person's ability to take turns, remember topics, or smile pleasantly (For an excellent outline of dementia and its impact, see Guendouzi & Savage, 2017). Helpful reviews on how conversation can support persons with dementia and techniques researchers often use are available. For example, Kindell, Keady, Sage, and Wilkinson (2017) discuss the beneficial exchange of information and social interaction in 50 conversation studies across four types of dementia, drawn from conversation analysis, collaborative storytelling, and other social and linguistic approaches.

Mikesell (2009, p. 138) illustrates beneficial potentials in her analysis of video-recorded conversations with a person diagnosed with frontotemporal dementia (FTD). A graduate student researcher worked with the person, his wife, and hired caretaker for roughly 50 hours, video-recording the conversations "over multiple instances and longitudinally to uncover recurrent patterns of discourse" (p. 159). The findings identified practices allowing researchers and family members to interact more successfully with persons who have FTD.

Speakers' cultural values are embedded in their discourse. For example, before we could collect data on whether a direct question-answer sequence affects walking (it does) in a New Zealand care home (Davis, Maclagan, Karakostas, Liang, & Shenk, 2011), we needed to learn about and participate in *karakia*, Maori prayers (Maori values, 2003). Similarly in the U.S., Hispanic, Asian, and non-Hispanic White family caregivers have been found to have different care practices (Miyawaki, 2016). For this reason, Brooke, Cronin, Stiell, and Ojo (2018) recommend that careworkers and health professionals receive training in culturally appropriate practices which include examining cultural perceptions of dementia and dementia discourse (see Schrauf, 2016). Researchers need to conduct culturally appropriate preparation for their prospective populations.

Identifying co-participants in conversations is key. Many of our consented conversations are collected by gerontology students allowed to visit and record specific people in memory care units (Hancock, Shenk, & Davis, 2009). Reliance on these students arose since professionally maintained residential sites seldom allowed us to record interactions between persons with dementia and staff or volunteer visitors. Insights and data collected from these student interactions have highlighted the need for intergenerational and volunteer training as well as the prevalence and problems inherent in question-answer routines, particularly with certain question types. The language used by people with different types of dementia can reveal how interactional, grammatical, pragmatic, or semantic differences arise during the course of a given condition.

The kind of question you ask may impede the kind of discourse you collect—and may even halt the talk from persons with dementia. For example, people with dementia not only take a longer time to answer questions; they take longer to answer some questions than others. Some questions are more difficult for them to answer than others. Tag questions (*You went to the mall, right*?) are easiest to answer although usually the least used, followed by *yes/no* and *so-prefaced* questions (*So, you have two sisters*?). The hardest questions to answer begin with *who, what, where, when, why,* or *how* (Davis, Maclagan, & Shenk, 2014). Persons with Alzheimer's dementia respond more slowly to episodic questions that ask for detailed memories (*what did you have for dinner last night?*) as opposed to semantic questions that ask for more general information (*What do you like to eat?*) (Small & Sandhu, 2008). Maclagan and Grant (2011, p. 85), reporting on the use of memory books by multilingual caregivers in New Zealand care homes, add that people collecting discourse should

> [a]void asking factual questions about the person's earlier life (*What work did you do?*). Instead, offer information for agreement (*I think you were a typist when you were younger*).

Practical Highlights for Caregivers

1. To initiate conversation and ease the burden of response, try statements, or tag questions: *You went to the mall, right?*
2. Avoid wh-questions (*when, where, who, how, why*) asking for specific information to prevent stressful or dangerous situations.

Reminiscence—stimulating participants to remember past events and experiences aloud—is widely practiced in collecting discourse and has a strong impact on coping and resilience among older persons (Meléndez, Fortuna, Sales, & Mayordomo, 2015): the well-known program of TimeSlips[1] (George & Houser, 2014; Vigliotti, Chinchilli, & George, 2018) fosters creative storytelling and other arts with its consented participants. Combining personal photographs and ethnographic interviewing (Sutton-Brown, 2014) often sparks language exchanges. Davis and Shenk (2015) find that videoclips from youtube.com or websites such as the American Memory Project (memory.loc.gov) can elicit personal reminiscence and prompt speakers to continue with more expansive comments and additional memories.

Practical Highlights for Caregivers

1. Choosing a variety of outside materials to stimulate both memory and talk may be helpful:
   (a) Photographs
   (b) Videoclips
   (c) Music
2. Consulting research findings using these techniques may help locate appropriate materials for persons in your care.

Activities such as interacting with laptops or photo-frames stuffed with moving photos or visiting museums or art galleries can often elicit recordable consented discourse. Astell et al. (2010) report good success using touch screen computers and specialized programs. Hamilton

[1] www.timeslips.org/; https://www.youtube.com/watch?v=9yxxbw7YIys.

(2011) conducted language analysis on video recordings of museum gallery tours for small groups of persons with dementia (see also Chapter 8). Group members were encouraged to share their responses to paintings with each other.

Practical Highlights for Caregivers

1. Visual stimulation activities engage persons with dementia and support memory, talk, and social engagement.
2. Small-group activities for persons with dementia can sustain rewarding social engagement.

Clinical testing can present difficulties for collecting dementia discourse unless language production or retention is part of the research project. Photos of famous people, tests of name recall, and wordless storybooks are all frequently used. Dijkstra, Bourgeois, Petrie, Burgio, and Allen-Burge (2002) outline screening for participant inclusion/exclusion criteria, their protocol for collecting language samples and their schema to assess or test for discourse features. Selecting the language test affords opportunities as well as issues: Sayegh (2015) reviews the impact of animal fluency and the Boston Naming Test across Hispanic and non-Hispanic White outpatients. For studies of the impact of aging on cognition and discourse production/comprehension, see Wright (2016): the various chapters offer a fine guide if language testing is desired.

Practical Highlights for Caregivers

1. Clinical testing protocols may offer some insight as to which materials—visual, written, audio, or video—would be appropriate for persons at different stages of particular dementia diagnoses.
2. Clinical testing protocols may also offer insights as to what kinds of activities might induce stress for persons with different conditions of dementia.

Collection Protocols

This section expands the questions from the section "Purposes" to help you design your research strategy for your purpose(s).

Identification of persons with dementia outside your own personal network of family and close friends is not easy. This challenge is in part due to the stigma still associated with the condition (Herrmann et al., 2018).[2] Unimpaired people often patronize, isolate, or discriminate against persons with dementia. For example, Johnson, Harkins, Cary, Sankar, and Karlawish (2015) identified that advanced age and beliefs that Alzheimer's was a mental illness would affect interpersonal interactions. Stites, Rubright, and Karlawish (2018) surveyed a random sample of U.S. adults asking probing questions such as whether they

> ...expected the person to have poor hygiene or neglect self-care – and the extent to which they expected people would be disgusted or repulsed by the person. (4)

Their findings concur with earlier work (see discussion section, Stites et al., 2018). Such stigma causes many older persons to hide their symptoms from their families, while many families hide their relative with dementia, fearing negative repercussions from friends and co-workers. Given these responses to stigma, identifying persons from whom to collect discourse without prior contacts to caregivers is difficult. Even with consent of the person or caregiver, without medical record access, analyses may be tentative, at best.

Recruiting persons may require you to visit residential sites as well as private homes and, consequently, entail that you speak with legal guardians or caregivers. We have found meetings helpful with facility directors and chaplains at professional residences, such as assisted living, memory care units, and nursing homes. They may put you in touch with legal guardians, and may also suggest specific residents. Take copies

[2]Please note that we are deliberately not calling such issues a disease, nor talking about stages, nor using deficit-based terminology.

of your Board of Ethics/IRB approvals and consent forms as you visit them, dementia support groups or respite care, adult day care centers, senior centers, or religious leaders. Recruiting African American persons may be especially difficult because of the history of medical mistreatment in the U.S. (Ighodaro et al., 2017). In South Asian communities, recognition of dementia has been observed to vary across age groups, perhaps contributing to delays in both identification and seeking care (Giebel et al., 2019). Watson, Ryan, Silverberg, Cahan, and Bernard (2014) review issues in recruiting for Alzheimer's clinical trials, including barriers for primary care providers and study partners who can report on a person's speech or behaviors. These barriers hold true for collecting all discourse.

Ethics regarding involvement of any kind with a vulnerable person requires examination and supervision. For research, every college, university, hospital, medical school, and most clinics report to Boards of Ethics or Institutional Review Boards. These Boards review proposed projects and researchers and go beyond assuring the anonymization and protection of personal and medical data. They ask hard questions about human rights protection. For example, how ethical is it to (1) use tracking devices with Global Positioning Systems (GPS) with community-dwelling persons who have dementia? (Landau & Werner, 2012) or (2) to monitor behaviors in order to develop, deploy, and evaluate assistive technologies that could extend independent living? (Meiland et al., 2017). Both projects could include interviews with persons who have dementia but are living independently at home: can they be assumed to handle the consenting process? The 2011 Dementia Ethics Research Project[3] developed by Alzheimer Europe, includes a discussion of potential burden and paternalism, adding that those with dementia

> …should not be treated like children or stereotyped as helpless. (Section 6)

[3]http://www.alzheimer-europe.org/Ethics/Ethical-issues-in-practice/2011-Ethics-of-dementia-research/The-dementia-ethics-research-project#fragment1.

Informed consent is the linchpin of any study involving the collection of discourse from persons who have dementia. The checklist furnished by the National Institutes of Health[4] lists the major concerns researchers should consider. For example, you must explain what kind of research you are doing and how the proposed participant will be involved to each legal guardian and, whenever possible, to each proposed participant. Although this sounds fairly simple, it is not.

How long will the person participate? Where? When? What benefits will accrue to the participant? How will confidentiality be maintained, and what risks or costs are foreseen? Can the participant stop at any time without any kind of penalty? The consent process must be conducted orally and in writing, and assurance that each person understands every part of the process is imperative. If you and the participant/guardian do not share the same language, you will need a qualified interpreter and an accurate translation of interactions and documents.

Even if persons with dementia are capable of signing the consent to indicate that they understand the project and their role in it, we advise having the approval and signature of legal guardians. Separate from your participant consent, this document needs to include your purpose, the location and duration of the project, how you are identifying and recruiting participants, the nature of your inclusion or exclusion of persons from the project, information about how you will protect the security of participants and their families, and how you will maintain the quality, security, and potential for others to use selections of anything you record. Involving caregivers of persons with dementia presents challenges of its own, but doing so preempts potential legal issues.

Caregivers—Finding and working with caregivers of persons with dementia may not be easy. As a case example, a study involving caregivers of U.S. veterans with dementia living in their communities (VA HSR&D Merit Award IIR HX001465) presented a variety of recruitment challenges. The electronic medical record of the Veterans Administration medical center

[4]http://nccih.nih.gov/sites/nccam.nih.gov/files/CR-Toolbox/Informed_Consent_Checklist_07-17-2015.docx.

generated a list of over 600 veterans diagnosed with dementia, but more careful screening found that those listed were often deceased or living in nursing homes or assisted living residences. A direct mail recruitment flyer sent to caregivers was followed by a round of phone calls to determine interest and eligibility. Often, 5–10 phone calls were needed to reach the primary caregiver. In addition, caregivers juggled multiple demands, either not living near their family members, complicated schedules, or, as observed in a home visit, caring for additional persons, such as grandchildren for working parents. Accordingly, the most frequent reason for declining study participation was a lack of time. Other researchers working from systems with electronic medical records may encounter similar issues.

While studies show interventions may also benefit caregivers (Piersol et al., 2017), descriptions of difficulties recruiting caregivers provide a cautionary picture (Leach, Ziaian, Francis, & Agnew, 2016; Morrison, Winter, & Gitlin, 2016). The majority of caregivers willing to participate are typically spouses over age 60, younger caregivers who often do not live with the person with dementia, and even children or grandchildren. One striking observation revealed caregivers whose caree had died were often the most committed to participating, perhaps hoping others could learn from their experience.

Equipment requires advance planning: you will need to include this information in the approval and consenting processes. While cameras and sound recording in current smartphones are excellent, they are not a substitute for professional equipment. Consult reviews of digital equipment for ease of use, quality of recording, and price (e.g., www.cnet.com).

Consider where you will store your recordings both for security and maintaining their quality. Academic and federal institutions often have password-protected, firewalled servers dedicated to storing research data on protected servers, a preferred venue of most Institutional Review Boards for such sensitive data.

Implications

When we study changes in dementia discourse, we are unwrapping more than syntax or lexicon or phonology, important though those are to the study of language variation and change. We are, rather, looking at human identity as speakers preserve their repertoire of social, cultural and personal identities through discourse, often in bits of rehearsed, twice-told tales featuring dialogue with speakers from the past (Davis & Maclagan, 2018, see recommended readings list). For this reason, each research protocol must be a thoughtful and careful look at the individuals behind the voices, the talk, we are collecting.

Practical Highlights

1. Identifying appropriate, willing persons with dementia can be challenging and time consuming.
2. Both institutions and caregivers can pose challenges to accessing persons with dementia.
3. Adherence to ethical practices and approval bodies such as IRB or Boards of Ethics is essential for research of persons with dementia; they are members of a vulnerable population whose conditions are still often stigmatized.
4. Planning a successful research protocol requires thoughtful consideration of every element from recording device, elicitation process, protection of persons involved and data security.

References

Astell, A., Ellis, M., Bernardi, L., Alm, N., Dye, R., Gowans, G., & Campbell, J. (2010). Using a touch screen computer to support relationships between people with dementia and caregivers. *Interacting with Computers, 22*(4), 267–275.

Brooke, J., Cronin, C., Stiell, M., & Ojo, O. (2018). The intersection of culture in the provision of dementia care: A systematic review. *Journal of Clinical Nursing, 27*(17–18), 3241–3253.

Davis, B., Maclagan, M., Karakostas, T., Liang, S., & Shenk, D. (2011). Watching what you say: Walking and talking in dementia. *Topics in Geriatric Rehabilitation, 27*(4), 268–277.

Davis, B., Maclagan, M., & Shenk, D. (2014). Exploring questions and answers between residents and caregivers. In H. Hamilton & W. Chou (Eds.), *The Routledge handbook of language and health communication* (pp. 344–361). New York, NY: Routledge.

Davis, B., & Shenk, D. (2015). Beyond reminiscence: Using generic video to elicit conversational language. *American Journal of Alzheimer's Disease and Other Dementias, 30*(1), 61–68.

Dijkstra, K., Bourgeois, M., Petrie, G., Burgio, L., & Allen-Burge, R. (2002). My recaller is on vacation: Discourse analysis of nursing-home residents with dementia. *Discourse Processes, 33*(1), 53–76.

George, D., & Houser, W. (2014). "I'm a storyteller!": Exploring the benefits of timeslips creative expression program at a nursing home. *American Journal of Alzheimer's Disease and Other Dementias, 29*(8), 678–684.

Giebel, C., Worden, A., Challis, D., Jolley, D., Bhui, K., Lambat, A., … Purandare, N. (2019). Age, memory loss and perceptions of dementia in South Asian ethnic minorities. *Aging & Mental Health, 23,* 173–182.

Guendouzi, J., & Savage, M. (2017). Alzheimer's dementia. In L. Cummings (Ed.), *Research in clinical pragmatics* (pp. 323–346). New York, NY: Springer.

Hamilton, H. E. (2011). At the intersection of art, Alzheimer's disease, and discourse: Talk in the surround of paintings. In P. Backhaus (Ed.), *Communication in elderly care* (pp. 166–192). New York, NY: Continuum.

Hancock, C., Shenk, D., & Davis, B. (2009). Integrating gerontology service-learning students as members of a research team. In P. L. Lim (Ed.), *Service learning and gerontology education* (pp. 171–184). New York, NY: Hampton Press.

Herrmann, L., Welter, E., Leverenz, J., Lerner, A., Udelson, N., Kanetsky, C., & Sajatovic, M. (2018). A systematic review of dementia-related stigma research: Can we move the stigma dial? *American Journal of Geriatric Psychiatry, 26*(3), 316–331.

Holden, T. R., Keller, S., Kim, A., Gehring, M., Schmitz, E., Hermann, C., … Kind, A. J. (2018). Procedural framework to facilitate hospital-based informed consent for dementia research. *Journal of the American Geriatric Society, 66*(12), 2243–2248.

Ighodaro, E. T., Nelson, P. T., Kukull, W. A., Schmitt, F. A., Abner, E. L., Caban-Holt, A., … Van Eldik, L. J. (2017). Challenges and considerations related to studying dementia in Blacks/African Americans. *Journal of Alzheimer's Disease, 60*(1), 1–10.

Johnson, R., Harkins, K., Cary, M., Sankar, P., & Karlawish, J. (2015). The relative contributions of disease label and disease prognosis to Alzheimer's stigma: A vignette-based experiment. *Social Science and Medicine, 143,* 117–127.

Kindell, J., Keady, J., Sage, K., & Wilkinson, R. (2017). Everyday conversation in dementia: A review of the literature to inform research and practice. *International Journal of Language and Communication Disorders, 52*(4), 392–406.

Landau, R., & Werner, S. (2012). Ethical aspects of using GPS for tracking people with dementia: Recommendations for practice. *International Psychogeriatrics, 24*(3), 358–366.

Leach, M., Ziaian, T., Francis, A., & Agnew, T. (2016). Recruiting dementia caregivers into clinical trials. *Alzheimer Disease and Associated Disorders, 30*(4), 338–344.

Maclagan, M., & Grant, A. (2011). Care of people with Alzheimer's disease in New Zealand: Supporting the telling of life stories. In P. Backhaus (Ed.), *Communication in elderly care* (pp. 62–89). New York, NY: Continuum.

Maori values and concepts (Tikanga). (2003). *Healthpoint.* Retrieved from https://www.healthpoint.co.nz/download,134977.do.

Meiland, F., Innes, A., Mountain, G., Robinson, L., van der Roest, H., García-Casal, J. A., … Franco-Martin, M. (2017). Technologies to support community-dwelling persons with dementia: A position paper on issues regarding development, usability, effectiveness and cost-effectiveness, deployment, and ethics. *JMIR Rehabilitation and Assistive Technologies, 4*(1), e1. Retrieved from https://rehab.jmir.org/2017/1/e1. https://doi.org/10.2196/rehab.6376.

Meléndez, J. C., Fortuna, F. B., Sales, A., & Mayordomo, T. (2015). The effects of instrumental reminiscence on resilience and coping in elderly. *Archives of Gerontology and Geriatrics, 60*(2), 294–298.

Mikesell, L. (2009). Conversational practices of a frontotemporal dementia patient and his interlocutors. *Research on Language and Social Interaction, 42*(2), 135–162.

Miyawaki, C. (2016). Caregiving practice patterns of Asian, Hispanic, and non-Hispanic White American family caregivers of older adults across generations. *Journal of Cross-Cultural Gerontology, 31*(1), 35–55. https://soi.oef/10.1007/s10823-016-9281-5.

Morrison, K., Winter, L., & Gitlin, L. (2016). Recruiting community-based dementia patients and caregivers in a nonpharmacologic randomized trial:

What works and how much does it cost? *Journal of Applied Gerontology, 35*(7), 788–800.

Piersol, C., Canton, K., Connor, S., Giller, I., Lipman, S., & Sager, S. (2017). Effectiveness of interventions for caregivers of people with Alzheimer's disease and related major neurocognitive disorders: A systematic review. *American Journal of Occupational Therapy, 71*(5), 1–10. https://doi.org/10.5014/ajot.2017.027581.

Prusaczyk, B., Cherney, S., Carpenter, C., & DuBois, J. (2017). Informed consent to research with cognitively impaired adults: Transdisciplinary challenges and opportunities. *Clinical Gerontologist, 40*(1), 63–73.

Rosato, M., Levey, G., Cooper, J., De Cock, P., & Devine, P. (2019). Factors associated with public knowledge of and attitudes to dementia: A cross-sectional study. *PLoS One, 14*(2), e0210543.

Sayegh, P. (2015). Neuropsychological language tests on dementia in English-speaking Hispanic and non-Hispanic White outpatients. *Applied Neuropsychology: Adult, 22*(6), 435–444.

Schrauf, R. W. (2016). *Mixed methods: Interviews, surveys, and cross-cultural comparisons*. Cambridge, UK: Cambridge University Press.

Small, J., & Sandhu, N. (2008). Episodic and semantic memory influences on picture naming in Alzheimer's disease. *Brain and Language, 104*(1), 1–9.

Stites, S., Rubright, J., & Karlawish, J. (2018). What features of stigma do the public most commonly attribute to Alzheimer's disease dementia? Results of a survey of the U.S. general public. *Alzheimer's & Dementia, 14*(7), 925–932. Advanced online publication. https://doi.org/10.1016/j.jalz.2018.01.006.

Sutton-Brown, C. (2014). Photovoice: A methodological guide. *Photography and Culture, 7*(2), 169–185.

Vigliotti, A. A., Chinchilli, V. M., & George, D. R. (2018). Enhancing quality of life and caregiver interactions for persons with dementia using timeslips group storytelling: A 6-month longitudinal study. *American Journal of Geriatric Psychiatry, 26*(4), 507–508.

Watson, J., Ryan, L., Silverberg, N., Cahan, V., & Bernard, M. (2014). Obstacles and opportunities in Alzheimer's clinical trial recruitment. *Health Affairs, 33*(4), 574–579.

Wray, A. (2016). Mechanisms of conflict and aggression in the dementia context. *Journal of Language Aggression and Conflict, 4*(1), 114–140.

Wright, H. (Ed.). (2016). *Cognition, language, and aging*. Philadelphia, PA: John Benjamins Publishing.

Recommended Readings

ADORE toolkit (Alzheimer's and Dementia Outreach, Recruitment, and Engagement Resources). (2019). *National Institutes of Aging*. Retrieved from https://www.nia.nih.gov/research/alzheimers-dementia-outreach-recruitment-engagement-resources.

Davis, B. (Ed.). (2005). *Alzheimer talk, text and context*. New York City, NY: Palgrave.

Davis, B., & Guendouzi, J. (Eds.). (2013). *Pragmatics in dementia*. Cambridge, UK: Cambridge Scholars Publishing.

Davis, B., & Maclagan, M. (2018). Represented speech. *Journal of Pragmatics, 130,* 1–15.

Guendouzi, J., & Mueller, N. (2006). *Approaches to discourse in dementia*. New York, NY: Psychology Press.

Hamilton, H. E. (1994). *Conversations with an Alzheimer's patient: An interactional sociolinguistic study*. Cambridge, UK: Cambridge University Press.

Kindell, J., Keady, J., Sage, K., & Wilkinson, R. (2017). Everyday conversation in dementia: A review of the literature to inform research and practice. *International Journal of Language and Communication Disorders, 52*(4), 392–406.

4

Why Use Interactional Data to Better Understand the Effects of Dementia?

Nicole Müller

Learning Objectives

By the end of this chapter, you will be able to:

- Consider the limitations of standard diagnostic and screening tests for dementia and cognition;
- Better understand and identify how dementia discourse within actual conversations demonstrates a person's abilities to competently negotiate real life interactions, even as the condition progresses;
- Appreciate and, subsequently, show appreciation of the person during conversations.

N. Müller (✉)
University College Cork, Cork, Ireland
e-mail: nicole.muller@ucc.ie

Linköping University, Linköping, Sweden

T. Stickle (ed.), *Learning from the Talk of Persons with Dementia*,
The Language of Mental Health, https://doi.org/10.1007/978-3-030-43977-4_4

Perspectives on Cognition

In the spring of 2018, the circumstance that U.S. President Donald Trump undertook a cognitive screening test was considered worthy of note in many media outlets not only in the U.S. but internationally. For instance, a headline in an Irish online news forum (www.thejournal.ie) ran, 'Could you pass the cognitive fitness test taken by Donald Trump this week?'[1]

The test in question was the Montreal Cognitive Assessment or MoCA (Nasreddine et al., 2005). The MoCA is a cognitive screening tool: A person taking the test is asked to complete a series of tasks that are arranged under the following headings: visuospatial/executive, naming, memory, attention, language, abstraction, delayed recall, and orientation. For instance, under the heading 'naming', the test-taker is asked to label line drawings of a lion, a rhinoceros, and a dromedary/camel. Under 'memory', the examiner reads a list of five words (four nouns, one adjective) and asks the test-taker to repeat the list twice. The MoCA is one of several widely used screening tools that are part of the test batteries employed to diagnose dementia and to quantify dementia severity. A further example is the Mini-Mental State Examination (MMSE) (Folstein, Folstein, & McHugh, 1975), which assesses a similar range of skills, with similar tasks. Such tests have several advantages: They are easy to use and score and don't require technology beyond paper and pencil. They are also quick to administer, and can be carried out by a wide range of professionals in many different health care contexts. They are also designed to be objective: The range of responses that are valid is very narrow, and therefore, very little room for interpretation or evaluation on the part of examiner is required (an answer is right or wrong, essentially). A discussion of the educational, cultural, and personal dimensions that potentially impact performance on such screening tests would lead us far beyond the confines of this chapter. What is important, however, is the perspective on cognition that underlies such tests, and, by a logical extension, we should ask the question what

[1] http://www.thejournal.ie/cognitive-test-donald-trump-3802251-Jan2018/.

a cognitive screening test can tell us about the functioning of a person with dementia.

The perspective on cognition embodied by the MoCA and MMSE (and others) is essentially modular in nature: Cognition is seen as composed of a set of discrete sub-skills, i.e., the DSM-5 uses the term 'neurocognitive domains' (American Psychiatric Association, 2013) that are separable from each other and can be measured in a discrete fashion. The composite score on MoCA or MMSE is used as a measure indicating the absence or presence of cognitive impairment, and in the latter case, an indication of severity. Any norm-referenced assessment, and cognitive screening tests are no exception, are designed to be as independent of context as possible. This also means that what is measured is, of necessity, abstract, in the sense that the task is performed for the sake of being tested, rather than for the sake of solving a problem that is an organic, natural part of daily life. Further, the sole focus of norm-referenced tests of cognition is on what an individual can do unaided. Thus, the perspective on cognition on which they are founded is not only modular but 'intracranial': Cognition is seen as the manipulation of abstract information that we do in the solitude of our own heads, without help from anything or anybody in our environments.

The modular, 'intracranial', but easily measurable (in terms of scores on standardized tests) approach to cognition is pervasive in clinical practice, not only in dementia-specific settings, but also in routine hospital encounters. At times it leads to an odd disconnect between so-called objective measurement and determination of cognitive impairment, and individuals' own perceptions. An example is the comparison of two cognitive screening tests administered in the context of acute hospital admissions, with report of subjective (that is, patients') memory complaint and informant report by Pendlebury and colleagues (Pendlebury, Klaus, Mather, de Brito, & Wharton, 2015). The authors found that the two cognitive screening tests (MoCA and AMTS, or the Abbreviated Mental Test Score, Hodkinson, 1972) correlated strongly with each other. However, they also found that there was only poor agreement between 'objective cognitive deficit' (as measured on MoCA and AMTS) and 'subjective memory complaint' and informant report, and that '39% [of patients] denying a memory problem had AMTS<9', the latter score indicating a cognitive deficit (Pendlebury et al., 2015, p. 1000). In addition, cognitive test scores did not match well with informant report (measured by means of a questionnaire), in that informant report both over- and under-identified cognitive decline as compared to the previous functioning.

Thinking Points

1. What is cognition?
2. How do we—as clinicians, researchers, persons—define cognition?
3. And, how do we measure and assess it?
4. Do cognitive processes occur only in one's own head, or do they extend into the world?

There is food for thought here along several dimensions[2]; what is most interesting for the present purposes is the reported mismatch: Measurement of cognitive deficit with standardized tools does not necessarily match the perceptions of the test-takers themselves or of familiar others. Pendlebury and colleagues used the question 'have you/has the patient been more forgetful in the past 12 months to the extent that it has significantly affected your/their daily life' (2015, p. 1001) in order to assess subjective memory complaint. If there is a mismatch between perception and test results, several possibilities arise. An obvious solution to the conundrum would be that people with memory decline may just not be aware of it. However, we know that in the early stages of, for example, Alzheimer's disease, and often before a diagnosis is made, many individuals are very much aware of their own declining faculties and how their lives are affected, which often leads to fear and frustration (Steeman, De Casterlé, Godderis, & Grypdonck, 2006). Another solution lies in another mismatch, namely that between what a

[2]Another dimension worth considering is the ranking of different types of knowledge, and that this might tell us of the status of patients versus practitioners: Objectively measured deficit is ranked higher in truth-value than subjective complaint (and a subjective complaint does not merit the term 'deficit'); a moral dimension is added by a substantial number of people with objectively measured deficit 'denying' that they have a memory problem.

decontextualized test measures (and how it does it), and the demands of daily life.

If we briefly reflect on how cognition works 'in the real world', or indeed 'in the wild' (Hutchins, 1995), we quickly realize that the default setting for people to solve the problems that life presents is to use whatever resources may be available, be that other people, artifacts and tools, or externalized and internalized practices. Management of our daily lives, our problem-solving, learning, intellectual growth (or degeneration), as well as our emotional and mental health (or ill-health), all happen during our interaction with other people.

We know that in dementia, cognitive faculties deteriorate and the 'staging' of cognitive decline in dementia by means of cognitive tests expresses the deterioration of unaided, decontextualized cognitive skills on tasks that are (deliberately) removed from any one individual's life, routines, or memories. And, without a doubt, we can remember, plan, evaluate, and problem-solve in the privacy of our own heads, but more typically and far more often, we do so, and learn to do so, in interaction with other people. Interaction represents continual challenges for cognitive skills (and deficits), as well as a tool box with which to meet those challenges. Given that human life is fundamentally interactive, a dialogic, interactive perspective arguably makes more sense if we want to learn how dementia affects the real lives of real people. Thus, a good starting point is to closely observe how people with dementia interact with other people, and how different interactions may help or hinder people with dementia, and their interaction partners, in coping with the demands of any one situation (see also Müller & Schrauf, 2014), including the demands posed by progressive neurological disease.

While an essentially context-free perspective on cognition is still (to my mind, unfortunately) pervasive and dominant in the clinical sciences, there is a growing body of research in cognitive science, philosophy and the social sciences that focuses on collaboration, context-embeddedness, embodiment and extension of cognitive processes beyond an individual's brain (see e.g., Meade, Harris, Van Bergen, Sutton, & Barnier, 2018, on collaborative remembering). Increasingly, such perspectives are also applied to living with dementia (see e.g., Blumen, 2018; Hydén & Kristiansson, 2018; Müller & Mok, 2018).

Thinking Points

1. Whether researcher, clinician, caregiver, or family member, think through your own concerns regarding the limitations of standard dementia diagnostic and assessment exams, particularly in light of your interactions with persons with dementia.
2. Whatever the context of those interactions, what details could provide a better understanding of the competency/ies of persons living with such conditions?

In the following section, I shall discuss some aspects of sense-making in interaction, and of situated, contextualized cognition, using examples from field observations and recorded conversations. Other chapters in this collection will address speech, language and interaction patterns (see Chapter 5 on pragmatic and discourse markers, Chapter 6 on syntactic errors, Chapter 7 on foregrounding competence through co-participant response), and present detailed discussions of interaction in dementia from a variety of perspectives and in different contexts (see Chapter 8, using place and objects for engaging interaction, Chapters 9 and 10 understanding dementia through emic reports, and finally, Chapter 11, enhancing the residential care experience).

Sense-Making in Interaction

The following example is an extract from a field note documenting observations in a nursing home in Louisiana (see Müller, 2009, for further details). Aimée is a nursing home resident with dementia; Todd was a graduate student and fellow field worker.[3]

[3]All names used in this chapter are pseudonyms.

Extract 1. (Field note: Aimée)

> Todd and I are sitting with a group of four residents around a circular table in the common room. [...] Aimée is sitting across from me; Todd is to my right [...] Aimée keeps glancing from Todd to me and back. She giggles quietly a few times. Todd refills my coffee cup and Aimée giggles again. She asks loudly, looking at me, 'is he your boyfriend?'

There are (at least) two perspectives from which we can approach interactions with people with dementia: We can look for deficits, or we can look for skills. From a deficit perspective, we might note that Aimée obviously does not remember what she has been told about Todd and myself on previous visits (difficulties laying down new memories; lack of recall of factual information). In addition, one could identify a deficit in reasoning (Todd is a generation younger than I am, so the likelihood of Todd being my boyfriend is probably slim), and indeed a deficit in social cognition: Asking two unfamiliar people without any preamble if they are romantically involved would be considered inappropriate. However, looking for skills we can note that Aimée is engaged in creating sense on the basis of the available evidence: There are two strangers, a young man and a not-so-young woman sitting opposite her at a table, they are friendly with each other, the young man performs a small service for the woman (by refilling her coffee). We don't know whether we are to take Aimée's question at face value, and if she is genuinely attempting to find out the relationship between the two strangers, or whether she is teasing them. (As an aside, we may note that a deficit-oriented perspective may risk missing genuine indications of humor.) In either case, her utterance demonstrates cognitive skills deployed in the moment of interaction in the sense that she is manipulating and interpreting perceptual (visual/auditory) information and uses it for interactive purposes.

Extract 2. (From conversation between Beatrice, Frances, Mary, and Rose; see Müller & Mok, 2014**)**

33.	M:	Hi Ms Beatrice.
34.	B:	Hello? (4.0) How y'all doin.
35.	M:	fine?=
36.	R:	=good thank you.
37.	B:	Y'all come visit?
38.	M:	[yeah.* ((*laughs*))
39.	R:	[mhm.*
40.	F:	come make a round to see me. I'm glad to have a little
41.		Company
42.	B:	She's your grandma?
43.	M:	no.=
44.	R:	=no.
45.	M:	no we're just visiting, (2.0) ((*chuckles*))
46.	B:	well y'all must know her then.
47.	M:	huh?

Extract 2 illustrates how Beatrice (B) uses questions to test hypotheses she forms about two young women she encounters chatting with Frances, who is Beatrice's friend, in Frances' room (see Müller & Mok, 2014, for a detailed analysis of the linguistic devices used in an extended interaction between these four participants). Both Beatrice and Frances are nursing home residents with dementia, and in the course of approximately two years of regular visits by myself and fellow field workers (here, Mary and Rose), did not show any indication of remembering factual information about us. However, as example 2 shows, Beatrice is curious about the visitors, and uses information that is available to her in the moment of interaction in order to formulate and test successive hypotheses about them. The first of these (line 37), confirmed by Mary and Rose, categorizes the strangers: They are visitors (as opposed to nursing home employees, or residents). The second hypothesis narrows down the category to a possible relationship between Frances and the visitors, and displays a combination of insight and lack thereof: On the one hand, the two visitors are evidently much younger than Frances, and thus Frances being their 'grandma' is feasible on the basis of observable age, as well as on the basis of social convention and practice: grandchildren visit grandparents. But it is not a likely relationship on the basis of observable ethnicity: Frances is African American, while Mary is Caucasian and Rose, Asian. Feedback from Mary and Rose leads Beatrice to abandon her previous hypothesis and she offers an alternative; if the two young women aren't Frances' kin, the only possible conclusion is that they know her.

This example illustrates three key processes of inquiry that are indicative of socio-cognitive competencies, interactive, and linguistic competencies: The use of contextual clues (Beatrice encounters two young strangers, chatting amiably with her friend Frances), the narrowing down of options on the basis of these clues, and the formulation and testing of hypotheses, in order to learn. This demonstrates not only that Beatrice has preserved skills of inquiry, but also the motivation, the drive, to learn. The evaluation of the skills and deficits of people with dementia more typically involves asking them questions and recording acceptable or unacceptable answers. In casual, day-to-day interactions, we can learn what sort of questions they ask, and thereby gain insight into what is important to them, and how they use information at their disposal to inquire into their.

Extract 3. (Field note: Orla's multimodal explanation)

[...] I've come to Orla's room to ask if she wants to come to the music session. [....] Orla looks at me for a few seconds without saying anything, then she grins. "Tá mé bodhar. Tá mé chomh bodhar le slios." ("I'm deaf. I'm as deaf as a post"). I have trouble understanding the final word, slis (it sounds like [ʃlis] to me), and I hesitate. She laughs, keeps looking at me. "Do you know what that is?"

NM: "[ʃlis], céard é sin?" ("a [ʃlis], what's that?")

Orla: "Níl sí ann anois." ("it's not around, now"). She mimes hitting something with a stick or the like, her right fist closed as if she's holding something, in a curved move

```
starting above her right shoulder and stopping
in front of her.
  NM: "Oh, slis. Ceart go leor." ("Oh, a slis
(rod, bat). Alright.")
```

Orla's first language is Irish, but she also speaks English fluently. She is a resident in a nursing home and has significant memory impairment consistent with dementia. She also, as she explains here, has hearing difficulties. I don't catch her explanation ('I'm as deaf as a post'), and she is aware of that, and mobilizes multiple resources to help me understand: She not only probes the source of my lack of understanding, but switches into English. I specify the problematic item, switching back into Irish, and she goes along with this. She then explains that the item in question is not 'around, now', which I interpret to mean, not in common use these days. She mimes hitting something with a stick or bat; one of the meanings of *slis* is rod or bat. She demonstrates considerably situated, context-embedded problem-solving abilities: She manages the repair of two potential sources of communication breakdown: my own lack of understanding, as well as what appears to be her own momentary word-finding difficulty (in either language): She addresses the former directly by asking me to confirm (lack of) comprehension and switching languages, and the latter by taking recourse to gesture. She thus demonstrates considerable situated, context-embedded problem-solving abilities, coordinating the use of two languages and non-verbal communication.

Practical Highlights

1. Paying close attention to how persons with dementia diagnoses use interactional resources allows us to see their abilities. These strategies include, but are not limited to, their use of question formation, word use, non-verbal cues of gesture and prosody.
2. More importantly, close attention to sophisticated employment of such resources can reveal what is of most interest to our co-participants with dementia diagnoses and, in turn, help us be better conversational partners who provide demonstrative concern for those concerns and for them as individuals.

Conclusion and Outlook

Some of the pioneering work on interaction in dementia was carried out in the 1990s and early 2000s—longer ago than most students remember! However, the studies conducted by, for example, Heidi Hamilton, Vaidehi Ramanathan, or Steven Sabat (see Hamilton, 1994; Ramanathan, 1997; Sabat, 2001) continue to inspire young researchers today, as does Tom Kitwood's work on dementia and personhood, which, while not primarily interested in studying interactions for their own sake, still has positive human interaction at its core (Kitwood, 1997). There is by now a very respectable body of work in this field, and it is fair to say that both research and clinical interest in interaction is still growing, and diversifying. In recent years, multilingual and mediated interactions, for instance in health care encounters, have gained increased attention (see e.g., Müller, 2017; Plejert, Antelius, Yazdanpanah, & Nielsen, 2015; Plejert, Lindholm, & Schrauf, 2017), as has the use of information and computer technology to support communication (e.g., Ekström, Ferm, & Samuelsson, 2017; Samuelsson & Ekström, 2019).

Interactional research permits us to focus on processes: on the ways people use language, or non-verbal means to make sense, in collaboration with others; how they remember together; how they enact identities, friendships; how they have arguments and misunderstandings. Closely examining interactions can give us insight in how people use contextualized skills, and how they draw on all the available resources in their environment. Therefore, examining interaction is both the antithesis, and therefore the necessary complement, to norm-referenced testing. While the latter can tell us about context-free skills and deficits, and permits us to draw broad-brush conclusions about, for instance, progressive deterioration of those skills across the population of people with various types of dementia, the former is necessary in order to gain insight into how people actually deal with the everyday challenges represented by cognitive deterioration. Dementia does not only affect the individual thus diagnosed: It affects an individual's whole social network, and it is by closely observing interactions that we can map the effects.

Interactional research on dementia can draw on an impressive tool box, as witnessed by the other chapters in this collection. Going forward, we need to draw on the tools we have, and the insights we have gained, to develop tools for clinical evaluation and intervention that holistically support living well with dementia. We also need to continue to advocate with professionals and policy makers in health care, eldercare, mental health, social work, speech-language pathology, and other disciplines that, in Tom Kitwood's words, the person (still!) comes first, and that enabling interactions, ranging from brief service encounters to diagnostic interviews to reminiscing, are at the core of living well—for all of us.

References

American Psychiatric Association. (2013). *Diagnostic and statistical manual of mental disorders: DSM-5™* (5th ed.). Arlington, VA: American Psychiatric Publishing Inc.

Blumen, H. M. (2018). Collaborative memory interventions for age-related and Alzheimer's disease-related memory decline. In M. Meade, C. B. Harris, P. Van Bergen, J. Sutton, & A. J. Barnier (Eds.), *Collaborative remembering: Theories, research and applications* (pp. 422–435). Oxford: Oxford University Press.

Ekström, A., Ferm, U., & Samuelsson, C. (2017). Digital communication support and Alzheimer's disease. *Dementia, 16*(6), 711–731.

Folstein, M. F., Folstein, S. E., & McHugh, P. R. (1975). Mini-mental state: A practical method for grading the cognitive stage of patients for the clinician. *Journal of Psychiatric Research, 12*(3), 189–198.

Hamilton, H. (1994). *Conversations with an Alzheimer's patient: An interactional sociolinguistic study*. Cambridge, UK: Cambridge University Press.

Hodkinson, H. M. (1972). Evaluation of a mental test score for assessment of mental impairment in the elderly. *Age and Ageing, 1*(4), 233–238.

Hutchins, E. (1995). *Cognition in the wild*. Cambridge, MA: MIT Press.

Hydén, L. C., & Kristiansson, M. (2018). Collaborative remembering in dementia: A focus on joint activities. In M. Meade, C. B. Harris, P. Van Bergen, J. Sutton, & A. J. Barnier (Eds.), *Collaborative remembering:*

Theories, research and applications (pp. 436–458). Oxford, UK: Oxford University Press.

Kitwood, T. (1997). *Dementia reconsidered: The person comes first*. Philadelphia, PA: Open University Press.

Meade, M., Harris, C. B., Van Bergen, P., Sutton, J., & Barnier, A. J. (Eds.). (2018). *Collaborative remembering: Theories, research and applications*. Oxford, UK: Oxford University Press.

Müller, N. (2009). Aging with French: Observations from South Louisiana. *Journal of Cross-Cultural Gerontology, 24*(2), 143–155.

Müller, N. (2017). 'Fear nó bean, a man or a woman?' Bilingual encounters in residential eldercare in Ireland. In C. Plejert, C. Lindholm, & R. W. Schrauf (Eds.), *Multilingual interaction and dementia* (pp. 57–73). Bristol, UK: Multilingual Matters.

Müller, N., & Mok, Z. (2014). "Getting to know you": Situated and distributed cognitive effort in conversations with dementia. In R. W. Schrauf & N. Müller (Eds.), *Dialogue and dementia: Cognitive and communicative resources for engagement*. New York City, NY: Psychology Press.

Müller, N., & Mok, Z. (2018). Memories and identities in conversation with dementia. In M. Meade, C. B. Harris, P. Van Bergen, J. Sutton, & A. J. Barnier (Eds.), *Collaborative remembering: Theories, research, and applications* (pp. 157–176). Oxford, UK: Oxford University Press.

Müller, N., & Schrauf, R. W. (2014). Conversation as cognition: Reframing cognition in dementia. In R. W. Schrauf & N. Müller (Eds.), *Dialogue and dementia: Cognitive and communicative resources for engagement* (pp. 3–26). New York City, NY: Psychology Press.

Nasreddine, Z. S., Phillips, N. A., Bédirian, V., Charbonneau, S., Whitehead, V., Collin, I., ... Chertkow, H. (2005). The Montreal Cognitive Assessment, MoCA: A brief screening tool for mild cognitive impairment. *Journal of the American Geriatrics Society, 53*(4), 695–699.

Pendlebury, S. T., Klaus, S. P., Mather, M., de Brito, M., & Wharton, R. M. (2015). Routine cognitive screening in older patients admitted to acute medicine: Abbreviated mental test score (AMTS) and subjective memory complaint versus Montreal Cognitive Assessment and IQCODE. *Age and Ageing, 44*(6), 1000–1005.

Plejert, C., Antelius, E., Yazdanpanah, M., & Nielsen, T. R. (2015). 'There's a letter called ef': On challenges and repair in interpreter-mediated tests of cognitive functioning in dementia evaluations: A case study. *Journal of Cross-Cultural Gerontology, 30*(2), 163–187.

Plejert, C., Lindholm, C., & Schrauf, R. W. (2017). *Multilingual interaction and dementia*. Bristol, UK: Multilingual Matters.

Ramanathan, V. (1997). *Alzheimer discourse: Some sociolinguistic dimensions*. New York City, NY: Routledge.

Sabat, S. R. (2001). *The experience of Alzheimer's disease: Life through a tangled veil*. Oxford, UK: Blackwell.

Samuelsson, C., & Ekström, A. (2019). Digital communication support in interaction involving people with dementia. *Logopedics Phoniatrics Vocology, 44*(1), 41–50.

Steeman, E., De Casterlé, B. D., Godderis, J., & Grypdonck, M. (2006). Living with early-stage dementia: A review of qualitative studies. *Journal of Advanced Nursing, 54*(6), 722–738.

Part II

Learning from the Talk of Persons with Dementia: Practical Steps for Doing and Applying Linguistic and Social Interactional Research

5

Signposts, Guideposts, and Stalls: Pragmatic and Discourse Markers in Dementia Discourse

Boyd H. Davis and Margaret Maclagan

Learning Objectives

By the end of this chapter, you will be able to:

- Describe the importance of "little words" like *but* and *so* in the speech of people with dementia;
- Identify pragmatic markers used by individuals with dementia in their interactions with others;
- Identify ways in which persons with dementia use these pragmatic markers.

B. H. Davis (✉)
UNC-Charlotte, University City Blvd, Charlotte, NC, USA
e-mail: bdavis@uncc.edu

M. Maclagan
University of Canterbury, Christchurch, New Zealand
e-mail: margaret.maclagan@canterbury.ac.nz

T. Stickle (ed.), *Learning from the Talk of Persons with Dementia*,
The Language of Mental Health, https://doi.org/10.1007/978-3-030-43977-4_5

Introduction

As dementia increases, working memory becomes less reliable and the methods that people with dementia once used in order to engage in conversation with others become less accessible. In particular, people with dementia may find it difficult to access the content words (nouns, verbs, adjectives, and adverbs) that provide the bulk of the meaning of what they want to say. Even when they do access these words, they may not use them in the appropriate context. However, they can usually still access many of the little words (grammatical words) like *but* or *so*. We don't *think* we pay attention to these words (though we do), and they are often neglected by researchers, but they can enable persons with dementia to keep their turns going or find their places in conversation. These words are often used as pragmatic markers: that is, their usage gives information to the hearer about how to interpret what the speaker is saying, and where the speaker is heading next: is it a new topic? A resumed topic? A question? An expanded story? A contradiction? The typical use of ***but*** is to suggest a contrast: *Mary had coffee* ***but*** *John had tea.* However, rather than indicating that something contrasting is coming, ***but***-final—***but*** at the end of a phrase—can signal that the person with dementia has lost their way in the conversation. ***But***-final may also indicate that the person with dementia wants to continue to talk. A person with dementia may use ***so*** with rising pitch and a longer pause to invite you, as a non-impaired person, to add information that could spark a recollection or a reaction from them. Another little word that is worth noticing is *well,* together with the phrase *you know,* and even the non-words *uh, um,* or *ah* that are often dismissed as merely marking a hesitation of some sort (Davis & Maclagan, 2020). Paying attention to little words pays off. And while our examples in this discussion are restricted to uses of ***but*** and ***so*** in English, other languages use other little words similarly: French *alors*, German *doch*, Swedish *ju*, or Japanese *–ne*.

Pragmatics is the study of the way people use language. These "little words" are pragmatic markers, or discourse markers (we do not make a distinction between these two terms). They allow people to establish common ground with their conversational partner, to signal that they are confused or to indicate that they disagree about something. Pragmatic markers can also be used to indicate a momentary loss of focus, or to hold the conversational floor while the speaker searches for a word or a phrase. People with dementia continue to use pragmatic markers to do all of these things, even as their dementia worsens. They also continue to use the conjunctions *but* or *so* which help to show how the conversation holds together. Maureen Littlejohn, for example, used both *but* and *so* as conjunctions to explain how her mother was able to go to college: "They'd paid as I probably told you, mother's way to go – go to college and – *but* she paid her brother's way to go to college, and he wouldn't go, and they wouldn't refund the money, *so* mother went in his place" (2013, interview with student P). However, like their use of silent pauses, filled pauses such as *uh* or *um,* or interjections, people with dementia often use *but* and *so* to substitute for some feature of conversational production that they can no longer access (see Davis & Maclagan, 2009, 2012, 2013, 2018, 2020). Talking to student LA who wanted to become a police officer, Littlejohn used both *uh* and *so* as pragmatic markers to hold her place in the conversation after she temporarily lost her way in her own story. She then used *but* rather than *however* to come back to what she wanted to say: "that will make promotions, I would think, come a lot quicker *uh so* like. *But,* you're still gonna have to pay your dues" (April 2013, with student LA).

Data

In this chapter we examine how the little words *but* and *so* are used by one speaker, "Maureen Littlejohn". Ms. Littlejohn was a white woman in her mid-eighties who lived in the memory care unit of an assisted living facility in the southeastern United States. Ms. Littlejohn consented to talk with students who were taking an introductory gerontology course at a nearby university (Hancock, Shenk, & Davis, 2009). Some of the students talked to her more than once as did the first author. The research received consent according to the IRB (Institutional Review Board) ethics regulations at the first author's university. At the start of the research, Ms. Littlejohn was able to consent to these conversations; as time went on, her niece renewed the formal consent, and Ms. Littlejohn continued to give her assent to each new conversation. The conversations took place over a period of six years.

In total, we recorded 39 conversations with Ms. Littlejohn. In this chapter, we refer to 24 of them. We use 16 conversations as we analyze her use of ***but*** and 18 to analyze ***so***. Our choice of conversation depended on the aims of our analysis. In order to analyze Ms. Littlejohn's use of ***but***, we chose one conversation with each of eleven students and five conversations with the first author. The conversations were spread evenly over the six years. For ***so***, the conversations we chose were again spread over the six years. However, this time we chose five conversations each with two of the students, four from the first author and one each from four students. The five conversations with each of the two students were all recorded within a short time period and allowed us to check Ms. Littlejohn's consistency of ***so*** usage. The first author is identified by her initials, BD, and the students are identified by "student" plus initials.

The conversations were all audio-recorded, with some of the later conversations with the first author being video-recorded. They were transcribed by HIPAA-compliant transcribers and donated to the Carolinas Conversations Collection (http://carolinaconversations.musc.edu). The speaker's name was changed to protect her privacy.

But

The word ***but*** is more complicated than we think. It can be used to signal several different meanings and can have several different functions in a conversation. Indeed, it occurs so frequently, we barely listen to it. Yet it guides our expectations for what comes next. We normally think of ***but*** as signaling the denial of someone's expectations and thus suggesting a contrast. The contrast may be explicit as shown in the following two sentences.

Larry is tall, ***but*** he's not good at basketball.
Petra is rich, ***but*** Jonnie is poor.

The contrast may also be implicit as in the following example from Fraser (2011, p. 33).

We started late, [=>We were going to arrive late] but we arrived on time.
But can also be used to offer a correction as in
My, your brother looks so much like you.
No, he is not my brother ***but*** my friend.

When we reviewed all 604 uses of ***but*** in the conversations with Ms. Littlejohn, we found that only 309 of them fell into the category of denial of expectations, 13 expressed an implicit contrast, 18 were used to offer a correction, and 9 were in clauses that were incomplete or interrupted. This means that only half of Ms. Littlejohn's uses of ***but*** actually signal the sort of contrast an unimpaired conversation partner might expect.

But in Initial Position

But can appear initially, medially, or finally in a sentence or utterance, with slightly different usage depending on its position. ***But-initial*** is used to manage telling a story, maintaining or resuming a topic, and to hold a turn while the speaker re-discovers what she wants to talk about. Figure 5.1 shows the uses for ***but-initial*** in the 16 conversations we

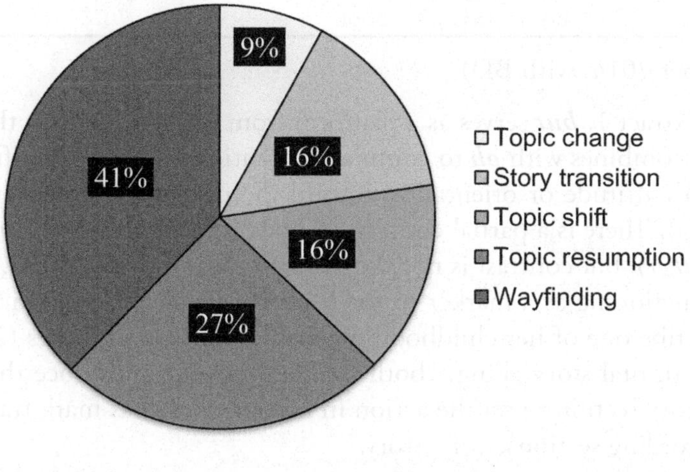

Fig. 5.1 *But*-initial usage in 16 conversations with Ms. Littlejohn (*Source* Authors)

used to analyze ***but***. Extract 1 gives an example of the use of ***but*** in initial position. Ms. Littlejohn is talking about her love of reading. She says that she inherited it from her parents, but more from her father than from her mother. Conventional punctuation is not used in this extract; rather it is set out to indicate pauses in Ms. Littlejohn's speech. One dash is equivalent to a pause of roughly half a second, two are equivalent to a whole second, and three are a second and a half, or a comparatively long pause.

Extract 1: Example of phrase-initial *but*

```
01.    --  my family
02.    --  my mother and father
03.    --  BUT oh I guess it's my father almost more than my
          mother
04.    --  have a
05.    -   I can remember
06.    --  we lived on a farm
07.    -   and I can remember
08.    -   him carrying a
09.    -   a book
10.    --- when he was
11.    --  whenever he was going out plowing
12.    -   and when he would stop to let the old horse rest
13.        for a w~ while
14.    --  he'd be reading a book
```

(October 2014, with BD)

In Extract 1, ***but*** serves as a platform from which to launch the story. It here combines with ***oh*** to command attention and "signal shifts in the speaker's attitude or orientation toward the discourse" (Redeker, 1991, p. 1153). There is a partial contrast in line 3 (*my father almost more than my mother*), but contrast is not the primary meaning of this ***but***. Rather, it is functioning as a marker to the listener that Ms. Littlejohn is about to describe one of her childhood memories. As Norrick notes (2001, p. 849), "In oral storytelling…both *well* and *but* can introduce the initial expository section to set the action in motion as well as mark transitions to succeeding sections…of a story."

But in Final Position

Local and Kelly (1986) say that ***but*** in final position can be a request for the partner to continue the conversation. Mulder and Thompson (2008) call ***but-final*** in English a "***hanging but***." This ***hanging but*** is losing its original grammatical force—it is grammaticalizing—so that it can be used as a discourse particle as well as a conjunction indicating contrast. The ***hanging but*** can often be a signal for turn transition, i.e., the person with dementia is indicating that the conversation partner should take over the conversation. In Ms. Littlejohn's usage, ***but-final*** is often a dual signal: she is trying to find her way as she has lost what she is trying to say to her partner and she will allow her partner either to take a turn or to offer a repair. In Extract 2, Ms. Littlejohn has been talking to BD about the fall colors. In her first turn (line 3), she uses conjunction ***but*** in its usual contrastive sense "***but*** there's not there's not too many" and then uses a final hanging ***but um*** (in line 4). Her conversation partner takes over the conversation and in her conversational turn moves the topic from autumn leaves to the birds that Ms. Littlejohn feeds and loves to observe. (<ooh> indicates a brief comment by BD; dots indicate a brief pause.)

Extract 2: Example of final *but* where Ms. Littlejohn has lost her way

01.	ML:	they have been beautiful this year . they have been
02.		just a beautiful shade of orange . <ooh> and they are
03.		they're still hanging on a little bit ***but*** there's not
04.		there's not too many ***but*** um -
05.	BD:	how about the birds? the birds have been attacking
06.		my bird feeder like crazy.
07.	ML:	have they really?

(November 2011, with BD)

Extract 3 occurred earlier in the same conversation. In this extract, Ms. Littlejohn is talking about inviting people home for dinner after church. She again uses conjunction ***but*** in its contrastive sense as she compares the ways things were in her childhood with how they are now (see lines 1 and 5). In line 12, her conversation partner acknowledges what they were talking about with <*right*>. *Right* is a general feedback term and Ms. Littlejohn could have carried on talking about bringing friends home to dinner (for example by talking about what her mother usually cooked) or she was free to change the topic. In line 13, she uses ***but*** **uh** followed by a pause of approximately one second (marked by - - in the text) indicating that she has lost the drift of what she was saying. Her conversation partner does not immediately step in, and Ms. Littlejohn summarizes this section of the conversation with a general comment about the "good old days" (lines 16–18).

Extract 3: Example of final *but* where Ms. Littlejohn has lost her way

01.	ML:	***but*** you couldn't let a kid do that now -
02.	BD:	no I don't think you can
03.	ML:	oh you couldn't
04.	BD:	and that's so sad
05.	ML:	i~ it really is sad <mm> ***but*** everybody we were truly
06.	-	neighbors
07.	-	more than neighbors uh because uh you might go
08.		to church and if you saw somebody there that you'd like to
09.		bring home with you for dinner you just ask 'em well come
10.		on home and we'll have dinner and uh
11.	-	it wasn't lunch or anything like that it was dinner
12.		<right>
13.	-	it was so **but uh**
14.	--	a lot of things about the good old days I wouldn't want
15.		to go back to
16.	-	***but*** then there are also lot of
17.	-	good old things that were
18.	-	uh would be pretty nice to have today

(November 2011, with BD)

Wayfinding

Wayfinding (like the clinical term *wordfinding*) is a term we have coined to signal when speakers have become lost in their own story or cannot immediately retrieve the gist of the conversation or the schema of a familiar event. According to Robin and Moscovitch (2017, p. 114),

> Gist refers to the central features of a particular episode (story line), and is distinct from schema, which refer to 'adaptable associative networks of knowledge extracted over multiple similar experiences'.

Extract 4 gives an example of Ms. Littlejohn losing the gist in one of her conversations. Again, a single dash represents a pause of roughly half a second and two dashes a pause of one second. The first author has just asked her if she watches reality shows on television. In line 1, Ms. Littlejohn answers the question and says that her life is not sufficiently interesting to be part of reality television. The pauses around ***but*** (line 3), together with the other frequent pauses, indicate that she has lost the gist of what she was trying to say.

Extract 4: Example of *but* indicating wayfinding, where Ms. Littlejohn has lost the gist of what she was saying

01.	-	I don't think they'll be knocking down the door to come and
02.		interview me here
03.	-	***BUT***
04.	-	no it's uh it's a good the employees are just
05.	-	you
06.	-	sit at the same table each time and
07.	-	it makes it easier on them to know that they're not having to
08.	-	stop and look around for where you're sitting today
09.	-	and um
10.	--	at a really basic one
11.	--	just keep on hanging in

(November 2012, with BD)

Topic Change and Topic Resumption

Sentence or phrase initial ***but*** is often used to change a conversation topic or to pick it up again. Bell (1998, p. 527) says that ***but-initial*** is "the 'discourse' or 'sequential' ***but***." He gives the following example, which he says is "a return to the main topic of discourse" (1998, p. 527):

A: We had a very nice lunch. I had an excellent lobster.
B: **But** did you get to ask him about the money?

Mentis, Briggs-Whittaker, and Gramigna (1995, p. 1055) say that, in order to be coherent, speakers must develop key ideas and be able to stay on the topic while expanding or elaborating these elements or ideas (cf. Hall, Lind, Young, Okell, & van Steenbrugge, 2018). Speakers must be able to take turns without being distracted and staying on topic involves cooperation from both of the speakers. In the following extracts, we see several kinds of ***but***-usage which enable Ms. Littlejohn to keep her story moving and on track. In Extract 5, Ms. Littlejohn is able to use ***But, oh*** (line 6) to start a new topic of conversation. With some encouragement from her partner, she produces a conventional discourse contrast to explain that modern buttermilk is not as good as it was when she was younger (line 17). (Dashes indicate brief pauses; non-speech is in square brackets [Laugh]; comments from her conversation partner are in italics in angle brackets < >.)

Extract 5: Use of *but oh* to change the topic of conversation

\- And they
\- and, and you couldn't go in and get it. You couldn't
bring back a little switch, because if you did
or you kept sended out until you got one
\- <don't go to the willow tree>. [*Laughs*]
\- Oh. Oh, dear. ***But, oh,*** I'll tell about good, old,
fresh buttermilk.
Let it get nice and cold. It was always good drinking. <Mm-hmm>
with lots of still with big globs of butter
all still wrapped in there.
\- <Yeah. Mm-hmm. It's hard to find in all the grocery stores
now>.
\- You know
\- well, the buttermilk that they, they call buttermilk
is just that it's aged. I don't think they do
anything particular to it,
but it's not like the old one

(April 2014, with student IAN)

In Extract 6, by contrast, her conversational partner is distracting, even as she tries to be encouraging. The partner talks just a little too much and introduces an unnecessary subtopic about tans. The sentence initial ***but*** (line 1) changes the topic and starts a new story about Ms.

Littlejohn's nephew, a "super" chef who arranged his job to be at the beach in the winter, and the mountains in the summer. The first two ***but***s (lines 1 and 7) are part of this story. The second sentence initial ***but*** (line 17) resumes the topic of how good he was at his job. The clause initial ***but*** in line 22 again brings the topic back to how good her nephew was as a cook. This is followed by a ***but anyway*** (line 27) which concludes this story by explaining that he was able to arrange his time by the seasons, the way he liked it. (Again the partner's utterances are in italics, in angle brackets < >; non-speech is in square brackets [laugh].)

Extract 6: Examples of Ms. Littlejohn's use of *but*

01. ***But*** his son, uh, Ken, went to the Waynesville Country Club
02. when he was just a kid for a, for a job, you know.
03. <Mm-hmm.>
04. And he got interested in cooking, and then he turned into
05. just a super chet
06. - chef. He's not
07. - you doing that as a living now, ***but*** he
08. - even years when he was working, he'd work in Florida in the
09. winter time and come home in Broughton, work at the
10. Waynesville Country Club in the summer time.
11. <Oh, that's the way to do it. Good weather all the time.>
12. *[Laughter]*
13. He was sure
14. - <He was tanned year round, I'm sure, wasn't he?> *[Laughter]*
15. - [*unclear*] the tans were pretty good, I'd say.
16. <Yeah. I bet. Country clubs.>
17. ***But*** *we* always, always liked to get invited to Ken's house
18. for Thanksgiving or Christmas dinner because [*sniffs*]
19. - <Mm-hmm.>
20. - now he would
21. - and he'd just, uh
22. - I reckon he's not working there, ***but*** he was an excellent cook.
23. <Yeah. Well, that must have been real nice.>
24. It was. Uh, and of course he was not married,
25. and he's still not married.
26. <Mm-hmm>.
27. Was a bachelor. ***But anyway***, to be able to work, uh, in Florida
28. in the winter time and then come home to Wayne[sville]

(April 2014, with student IAN)

But—Summary

But is multifunctional and that multifunctionality is exploited by the speaker with dementia. We earlier noted its use for denying expectations or offering contrasts in 349 out of a total 604 uses. The remaining 255 were typically used to open or to close a topic. ***But*** can appear initially, medially, or finally in a sentence or utterance, with slightly different usage depending on its position. ***But*** is especially important for both topic change and topic maintenance. Like other pragmatic markers such as *well*, it can also be used to hold the floor. Depending on the context, ***but*** in final position can either be used to hold the floor while the speaker sorts out how to continue or else as a signal to the conversation partner to take a turn. The length of the following pause is typically what disambiguates the two meanings.

Thinking Points

1. The use of ***but*** does not necessarily mean that the speaker with dementia is objecting to what the conversation partner has said.
2. Frequently, ***but*** is a floor holder while the speaker with dementia is preparing to continue to speak.

So

So is a word that is used often and in multiple ways. ***So*** can be used initially, medially, and finally in an utterance but with different meanings. When ***so*** is used in medial position, it is most often a conjunction rather than a pragmatic marker. Typically, ***so*** in medial position means something like "***so*** consequently" or "as a result":

Mary needed cauliflower, ***so*** she went to the market.

Rapunzel saw no staircase available, ***and so*** she slid down her long braids.

In the following brief extract, Ms. Littlejohn uses ***so*** as a medial conjunction as she explains to one of the students that her niece organizes everything she needs for the residence where she lives:

> my - this one niece in particular is just uh she was you know she just handles any any bills any business anything that needs <Hmm> to be done ***so*** I'm about as stressless as can be [laughter].
>
> (February 2010, with student L)

So in Initial Position in an Utterance

When ***so*** is used in initial position (called ***so***-initial or ***so***-preface) it can introduce an utterance that summarizes what has been said or done previously. It often serves to return the conversation to the main topic (Davis, 2005, p. 136; Raymond, 2004, p. 186). If the conversation partner uses it, ***so***-initial frequently acts as an indirect question or a request for expansion. When used by the speaker with dementia, ***so***-initial is often an allusion to prior talk and may combine with additional markers to act as place holders or as some flavor of evaluation. In the following extract, Ms. Littlejohn is explaining how her handmade basket for carrying eggs was woven to have two compartments. She uses a string of pragmatic markers ***so, but, anyway*** to combine a semi-modest demurral with an overall evaluation of her basket making:

> the reason for that is you could put half your eggs on this side and half on that and distribute the weight and run less risk of cracking them. ***So but anyway***, I enjoyed making them.
>
> (Fall 2009, with students A and C)

In Extract 7 (below), a ***so***-preface is used in two slightly different ways. In line 1, L, the partner, begins with a ***so***-prefaced question as she probes further in their discussion of meals at the residence. Ms. Littlejohn's ***So uh*** in line 7 prefaces an evaluative conclusion that is designed to be reassuring and, with any luck, to close the topic "for sure."

Extract 7: Examples of *so* in initial position in an utterance

01.	L:	***So*** do you get to select what food you want to eat every day?
02.	ML:	No, well I guess to some degree you know you do uh but uh
03.		If there's something you really really don't like
04.		or what have you or if there's something you really don't like
05.		of course they'll always fix you a cheese sandwich.
06.	L:	<Hmmm.> [*this is an approving hmmm with a falling contour*]
07.	ML:	***So uh*** we don't go hungry for sure

(February 2010, with student L)

Later in the same conversation, Ms. Littlejohn uses a ***so***-preface to close one topic and move to a new one. She has been talking about how she moved around the country, changing jobs as a respiratory technician whenever she wanted some new training or opportunities in her work. Her ***so and then*** starts a new variation on the topic of travel, focusing on retirement-travel rather than travel for work:

> ***So and then*** after my husband retired we bought us a uh truck and what's called a fifth wheel trailer.
>
> (February 2010, with student L)

In the same conversation, she similarly uses ***so but uh*** to move from a description of her life to her bird feeder and the new topic of how much she enjoys watching the birds outside her room:

> ***So but uh*** and even on dreary days like this it's you know can still be have my bird feeder out there just outside the window.
>
> (February 2010, with student L)

So in Final Position in an Utterance

So at the end of an utterance, or ***turn-final so***, often closes more than a turn, it closes a whole topic. Koivisto and Voutilainen (2016, p. 239) comment that in addition to "projecting a conclusion," the ***turn-final so*** can be treated as an invitation to the conversation partner to draw an inference and ask questions or expand the topic. In Extract 8,

Ms. Littlejohn has been talking to students A and C about yard sales and the treasure you can sometimes find there. In line 5, her ***turn-final so*** indicates that she has said all she wants to on the topic. Student C picks this up in line 6 with a concluding saying (‘*another man's junk is another man's treasure*’). In line 7, Ms. Littlejohn agrees emphatically (‘*You're absolutely right*’) and then concludes the section with a self-deprecating comment (‘*I never found the treasures*’). The laughter confirms that all three participants know that they have finished this section of the conversation. The students appropriately turn the conversation to the new topic of baskets that Ms. Littlejohn made and has on display in her room.

Extract 8: Example of turn-final *so* used to close a topic

01.	ML:	There are just wonderful little old antiques
02.		- not so little price wise but that doesn't seem to go down
		- but you can pick up
03.		- in yard sales it's just amazing
04.		what you can find in them
05.		- ***so***
06.	C:	they say another man's junk is another man's treasure
07.	ML:	That you're absolutely right, that is that's for sure.
08.		The only trouble is I usually ended up with junk, [*all laugh*]
09.		I never found the treasures. [*all laugh*]

(Fall 2009, with students A and C)

In the following brief extract, Ms. Littlejohn has been explaining to student LA that staff in the residence are on duty all the time. Her ***turn-final so*** indicates that she has said all she wants to about daily life at the residence. The student realizes that the topic is finished, but instead of completely changing the topic, he asks whether Ms. Littlejohn has been on any interesting outings from the residence recently. (LA's comments are in italics in angle brackets < >.)

they're all out there at the desk, they can keep track all day and night to see <*Watch out for you. Yeah*>. [laughing] To watch out. To see if I'm minding my own business, you know. [laughing] ***So.*** <*Ya'll - Ya'll done anything lately? Ya'll been anywhere or?*>

(April 2013, with student LA)

Interestingly, ***so*** is also used in an extender in the phrase, ***and so on.*** Extenders are often found at the end of a list, either long or short, to suggest there are more items. They also can serve as an invitation to the conversation partner to fill the list with more items (Maclagan, Davis, & Lunsford, 2008). The following example is one of the fourteen times Ms. Littlejohn used this phrase in the same conversation with LA:

> it still is an area that people they just attract a lot of visitors in the summer time you know is come and just be a part of the crafts and art shows. <*Hmm.*> ***And so on.***
>
> (February 2010, with student L)

So–Summary

Ms. Littlejohn used ***so*** relatively frequently in her conversations. In Fig. 5.2, the dark bars show the number of times she used ***so*** as a pragmatic or discourse marker in the 18 conversations we analyzed. It is clear that she used pragmatic marker ***so*** in each of the conversations. However, because the conversations differed in length, a simple direct comparison of ***so*** usage is not particularly meaningful. The light bars show how many times Ms. Littlejohn used ***so*** as a pragmatic marker for every 1000 words spoken by both speakers in the conversation. She used ***so*** sufficiently frequently that even in the conversations where she used it least often, Ms. Littlejohn still produced almost two discourse marker ***so*** per 1000 words.

Ms. Littlejohn used ***so*** in many other ways, apart from her use of it as a discourse or pragmatic marker. Because this chapter is focusing on the role of ***but*** and ***so*** as pragmatic or discourse markers that are used to guide the conversation, we have ignored her use of it in other ways, such as an emphasizer: *I'm so tired!* In Extract 9 from October 2010, she used ***so*** in three different ways in the one conversational turn with student B. In line 1, she uses initial ***so*** as a summary of the previous section of the conversation about her niece and the dog Izzy, which Ms. Littlejohn loves to see. In line 2, she uses ***so*** in its common sense as an intensifier—Izzy is ***so*** gentle. In line 4, she again uses initial ***so*** as a summary, and in line 5, she uses final ***so*** to hand the conversational topic over to the student.

Extract 9: Three different uses of *so* in one conversational turn by Ms. Littlejohn

01.	***So*** she's going to come over and bring Izzy. - 'cause he he's just
02.	- - a great big old - - awkward mutt but he's just ***so*** - - ***so***
03.	gentle in his awkwardness kind of makes sense - and she just he's
04.	Izzy goes pretty much with her ***so*** she's coming by to see me and
05.	bring Izzy ***so***

(October 2010, with student B)

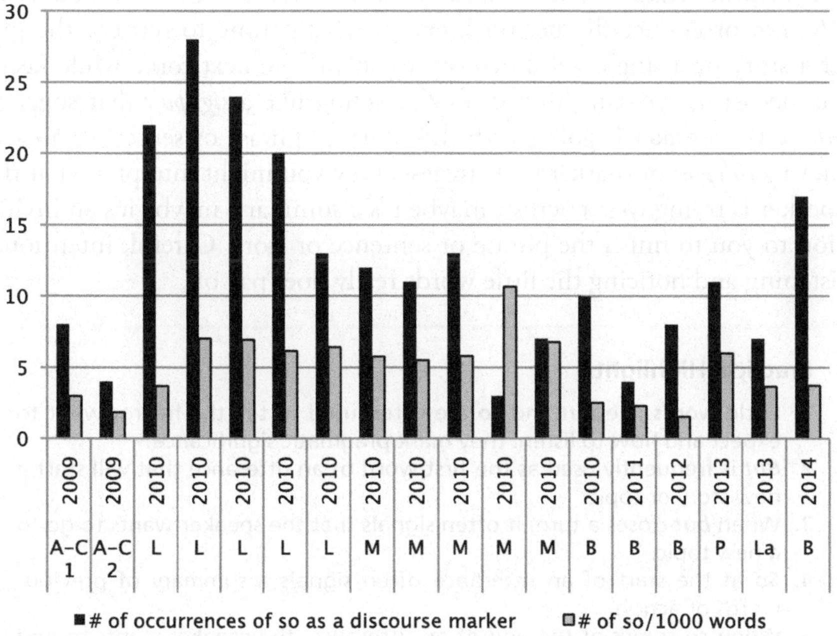

Fig. 5.2 The raw number of occurrences of ***so*** as a discourse marker together with its frequency as a discourse marker per 1000 words (*Source* Authors)

Thinking Points

1. Be aware that ***so*** can be used as a discourse marker as well as an emphasizer.
2. ***So*** at the end of an utterance can be used to hand the topic over to the unimpaired speaker.

Summary

In this chapter, we have analyzed the way that Maureen Littlejohn, a woman with dementia, used the "little words" ***but*** and ***so*** as pragmatic or discourse markers to help structure her conversations over six years. If the chapter has a message, it's that active and careful listening may be your most important task until you can figure out how your conversational partner who has dementia is using little words to signal the direction of the communication. *Stalls*—usually some variation or combination of *uh, um*, or *er*—let the person literally stall for time to retrieve the gist of a story or a single word or even to "plan" the next topic while keeping her turn. We can think of ***but*** as acting like a *signpost* that suggests where the speaker is going with this story or phrase or sentence. ***So*** acts like a *guidepost* or marker that suggests how you might interpret what the speaker is trying to get across: maybe it's a summary, maybe it's an invitation to you to finish the phrase or sentence or story. Careful, intentional listening and noticing the little words really does pay off.

Practical Highlights

1. Little words like ***but*** and ***so*** are often used to tell the hearer what to expect and how to listen: they mark pragmatic significance.
2. ***But*** is frequently used as the first word of an utterance that will start a new story or topic.
3. When ***but*** closes a turn, it often signals that the speaker wants to go to a new topic.
4. ***So*** at the start of an utterance often signals a summary of previous words or action.
5. When ***so*** comes at the end of an utterance, the speaker wants to end that topic.
6. Paying attention to little words like ***but*** and ***so*** will help you to keep track in a conversation with someone who has dementia.

Activity

- ***Go-aheads*** **and** ***quilting*** are useful techniques to keep a conversation going with a person with dementia (see Davis, Maclagan, & Shenk, 2014).
- **A** ***go-ahead*** is a two-syllable phrase like *Uh-huh, Mmm-hmm*, or *Oh really! Go-aheads* are used to encourage your conversation partner to carry on with what she was saying. *Go-aheads* need to be two syllables (*mmm-hmm* rather than *mmm*) so the person with dementia has a better chance of hearing them. Most of us use these phrases automatically; when you are talking with someone who has dementia, it can be helpful if you use them slightly more often.
- ***Quilting*** allows you to help the person with dementia tell a story. As you are talking, you may notice that your conversation partner uses a particular word or phrase. Ms. Littlejohn, for example, often talked about taking apples to school. When she mentioned *apples*, her conversation partner would say something like "you always took apples to school" with a rising pitch, and then pause in a way that invited her to continue. Over time, more details of her love of apples emerged in the conversations.

Activity: Practice with another student, co-worker, carer, fellow researcher to learn how to use ***go-aheads*** or ***quilting*** in your interactions.

References

Bell, D. (1998). Cancellative discourse markers: A core/periphery approach. *Pragmatics, 8*(4), 515–541.

Davis, B. (2005). So, you had two sisters, right? In B. Davis (Ed.), *Alzheimer talk, text and context* (pp. 128–145). New York, NY: Palgrave.

Davis, B., & Maclagan, M. (2009). Examining pauses in Alzheimer's discourse. *American Journal of Alzheimer's Disease and other Dementias, 24*(2), 141–154. https://doi.org/10.1177/1533317508328138.

Davis, B., & Maclagan, M. (2012). Stylistic usage of pragmatic markers and habituated pauses: Performative functions retained by older speakers. In P. G. Blitvich & M. Macaulay (Eds.), *Pragmatics and context* (pp. 73–96). York, Canada: Antares.

Davis, B., & Maclagan, M. (2013). "Talking with Maureen": Extenders, and formulaic language in small stories and canonical narratives. In R. W. Schrauf & N. Müller (Eds.), *Dialogue and dementia: Cognitive and communicative resources for engagement* (pp. 87–120). New York, NY: Psychology Press.

Davis, B., & Maclagan, M. (2018). Represented speech in dementia discourse. *Journal of Pragmatics, 130,* 1–15.

Davis, B., & Maclagan, M. (2020). UH as a pragmatic marker in dementia discourse. *Journal of Pragmatics, 156,* 83–89. https://doi.org/10.1016/j.pragma.2018.12.005.

Davis, B., Maclagan, M., & Shenk, D. (2014). Exploring questions and answers between residents and caregivers. In H. Hamilton & W. Chou (Eds.), *The Routledge handbook of language and health communication* (pp. 344–361). New York, NY: Routledge.

Fraser, B. (2011). The sequencing of contrastive discourse markers in English. *Baltic Journal of English Language, Literature and Culture, 1,* 29–35.

Hall, K., Lind, C., Young, J. A., Okell, E., & van Steenbrugge, W. (2018). Familiar communication partners' facilitation of topic management in conversation with individuals with dementia. *International Journal of Language & Communication Disorders, 53*(3), 564–575. https://doi.org/10.1111/1460-6984.12369.

Hancock, C., Shenk, D., & Davis, B. (2009). Integrating gerontology service-learning students as members of a research team. In M. Moore & P. Lan Lin (Eds.), *Service-learning in higher education: Paradigms and challenges* (pp. 171–184). Indianapolis, IN: University of Indianapolis Press.

Koivisto, A., & Voutilainen, L. (2016). Responding to what is left implicit: Psychotherapists' formulations and understanding checks after clients' turn-final Että ("That/So"). *Research on Language and Social Interaction, 49*(3), 238–257.

Local, J., & Kelly, J. (1986). Projection and 'silences': Notes on phonetic and conversational structure. *Human Studies, 9*(2), 185–204.

Maclagan, M., Davis, B., & Lunsford, R. (2008). Fixed expressions, extenders and metonymy in the speech of people with Alzheimer's disease. In S. Granger & F. Meunier (Eds.), *Phraseology: An interdisciplinary perspective* (pp. 175–186). Amsterdam & NY: John Benjamins.

Mentis, M., Briggs-Whittaker, J., & Gramigna, G. (1995). Discourse topic management in senile dementia of the Alzheimer's type. *Journal of Speech and Hearing Research, 38*(5), 1054–1066.

Mulder, J., & Thompson, S. (2008). The grammaticization of *but* as a final particle in English conversation. In R. Laury (Ed.), *Crosslinguistic studies of clause combining: The multifunctionality of conjunctions* (pp. 179–204). Amsterdam: John Benjamins.

Norrick, N. (2001). Discourse markers in oral narrative. *Journal of Pragmatics, 33*(6), 849–878.

Raymond, G. (2004). Prompting action: The stand-alone 'So' in ordinary conversation. *Research on Language and Social Interaction, 37*(2), 185–218.

Redeker, G. (1991). Linguistic markers of discourse structure. *Linguistics, 29*(6), 1139–1172.

Robin, J., & Moscovitch, M. (2017). Details, gist and schema: Hippocampal–neocortical interactions underlying recent and remote episodic and spatial memory. *Current Opinion in Behavioral Sciences, 17,* 114–123.

Recommended Readings

Davis, B. H., & Maclagan, M. (2017). Language issues in multilingual dementia care: a fast-growing issue. *The Linguist, 56*(4), 26–27. Retrieved from https://thelinguist.uberflip.com/the-linguist-archive/the-linguist-56-4-august-september-2017.

Davis, B. H., & Maclagan, M. (2018). Narrative and aging: Exploring the range of narrative types in dementia conversation. *European Journal of English Studies, 22*(1), 76–90.

Davis, B. H., & Maclagan, M. (2018). Represented speech in dementia discourse. *Journal of Pragmatics, 130,* 1–15.

Davis, B. H., Maclagan, M., & Shenk, D. (2016). The silent violence of marginalization and teasing in dementia care residences. *Journal of Language Aggression and Conflict, 4*(1), 35–61.

Davis, B. H., Maclagan, M., & Wright, J. (2013). 'Aw, so, how's your day going?': Ways that persons with dementia keep their conversational partner involved. In B. H. Davis & J. Guendouzi (Eds.), *Pragmatics in Dementia Discourse* (pp. 83–116). Newcastle upon Tyne, UK: Cambridge Scholars.

Guendouzi, J., Davis, B. H., & Maclagan, M. (2015). Listening to narratives from people recently diagnosed with dementia. *Transactions in Language Disorders, 35*(3), 237–257.

Guendouzi, J., Williams, M. J., & Manasco, H. (2010). Mental health literacy: The influence of professional and public discourses on Allied Health students' perceptions of dementia. *Journal of Interactional Research in Communication Disorders, 1*(1), 119–133.

Hamilton, H. E. (2008). Narrative as snapshot: Glimpses of the past in Alzheimer talk. *Narrative Inquiry, 18*(1), 53–82.

McCaghren, K., & Guendouzi, J. (2011). "First impressions": Perceptions of communicative abilities in people with traumatic brain injury. *Journal of Interactional Research in Communication Disorders, 2*(1), 101–129.

6

Making Sense of Syntactic Error in Conversations Between Persons with Dementia and Their Non-impaired Co-participants

Trini Stickle and Anja Wanner

Learning Objectives

By the end of this chapter, you will be able to:

- Recognize common syntactic errors correlated with dementia progression;
- Recognize common linguistic and interactional symptoms for several dementias;
- Identify co-participant strategies that may facilitate conversation, including with those experiencing severe linguistic losses;
- Respond to persons experiencing such losses in ways that they perceive sense of identity and dignity during interaction.

T. Stickle (✉)
Western Kentucky University, Bowling Green, KY, USA
e-mail: trini.stickle@wku.edu

A. Wanner
University of Wisconsin-Madison, Madison, WI, USA
e-mail: awanner@wisc.edu

T. Stickle (ed.), *Learning from the Talk of Persons with Dementia*,
The Language of Mental Health, https://doi.org/10.1007/978-3-030-43977-4_6

Introduction

Many people suffer no significant loss of linguistic abilities as they age, yet others experience great language loss as the result of age-related degeneration due to any number of neurocognitive diseases. These changes are primarily brought on by dementia, a syndrome caused by any number of progressive disorders that affect memory, thinking, communication, and the ability to perform everyday activities (American Psychiatric Association, 2013). The degenerations in neurostructures associated with dementia lead to a progressive decline in memory and language quality, both of which effect persons' facility to easily participate in everyday conversations. The cumulative effect, then, robs persons of their perceived role as a productive conversation participant, a vital part of their identity. This inability to communicate with fellow human beings due to disruptions among memories, retrieval of words, and disruptive or disjointed syntax can cause persons diagnosed with dementia to "withdraw from social activities for fear of being seen as a burden to others or as failures when their disabilities come to show themselves" (Ryan, Bannister, & Anas, 2009).

In this chapter, based on transcriptions of actual conversations with individuals diagnosed with dementia, we look at some of the linguistic constructions used and at how those constructions, particularly in regard to syntactic non-fluency, can have observable effects on conversation. We then highlight the application of participant strategies that seem to allow continued, productive interaction. After an overview of our previous work in this area, we present a case that illustrates common but relatively benign difficulties persons diagnosed with dementia may display within conversations. Next, we examine two persons with severely impaired linguistic abilities and the interactional strategies employed by their co-participants that seem to allow the persons with dementia a small window to use language effectively and to participate productively in their respective conversations. Our analysis shows that when co-participants respond to impaired syntax as making sense or completing a syntactic–semantic action, participants with dementia may use these cues to employ better communicative language (if only briefly). From these observations, we examine co-participants' linguistic and interactional choices as possible models of (best) communication practices applicable to home, clinic, and research settings.

Preliminaries: Our Participants and Methods of Discovery

The short analyses we present in this chapter are part of ongoing work in which we employ a mixed analytic approach that combines insights from corpus-based syntactic analysis with interactional methods, which we believe brings forth the salience of our participants' online performance within the conversation data. In that work, we conduct a close syntactic analysis of the verbal patterns during actual conversations produced by the persons residing in assisted living facilities who have a diagnosis of dementia. This allows us to describe two levels of linguistic production. On one level, we characterize their linguistic behavior in terms of grammatical structures, particularly in terms of adherence to normative and/or standard usage. Specifically, grammatical pattern types and frequencies are compared to patterns of usage recorded in benchmark corpus studies that capture the syntactic patterns and errors of (presumably) non-impaired persons (Biber et al., 1999). The reason behind this is that we want to see if potential difficulties in co-constructing a conversation might have their root in difficulties in accessing syntactic patterns. We pay particular attention to verbal constructions that require knowledge of (and access to) the syntax-semantics interface. At the conversational level, we describe how utterances are fitted to the emerging conversation as well as responded to by the co-participant(s). We closely follow both the fittedness (i.e., appropriateness and correctness) and production (i.e., original verbal forms versus reuse of a co-participant's linguistic resources) selected by each participant to better understand the use of linguistic resources in relation to the progression of talk (and vice versa). We also look at how topic development and communication actions (e.g., question-answer, compliment-response) are more or less successfully completed as evidenced by the participants themselves. During our analysis, the grammaticality of the utterances are coded in terms of "error" or "no error"; however, more importantly, the second level of analysis examines whether "errors" or usages that deviate from the norm seem to create trouble for the co-participants as evidenced by overt cues such as clarification questions (e.g., "what?" or "huh?") or difficulty in keeping up the conversation. These data are quantitatively and qualitatively tracked. Through this two-level analysis, a more complete interactional portrait of persons who are diagnosed with dementia emerges. The extracts that we discuss later in this chapter are not so comprehensively reported on; rather, we highlight issues of more practical relevance to the mission of this book.

The primary data for our work consist of audio-recorded conversations of face-to-face talk between twenty dyads, each comprised of a person diagnosed with dementia of the probable Alzheimer's type and a non-impaired co-participant. The data are part of the Carolinas Conversation Collection (CCC), a specialized web portal housed at the Medical University of South Carolina (Pope & Davis, 2011). The CCC contains collections of conversational interviews with people who are 65 or older, some of whom have been institutionalized due to a diagnosis of dementia. Full disclosure of the participants' medical records, including tests and comorbidities, is not required to be part of the CCC research database. While we would prefer to have complete disclosure of each person's demographic information, comorbidities, and the results of diagnostic exams, these conversational interviews do provide a window into the daily interactions that persons institutionalized with a dementia diagnosis engage in as they interact with non-intimate, non-impaired persons—a situational setting that is not all that different from interactions with medical professionals or caregivers.

Normalized transcripts provided through the CCC portal were subsequently converted to meet conversational analytic standards (Atkinson & Heritage, 1984; Jefferson, 2004). Names and identifying information were permanently removed from the audio recordings. Pseudonyms were ascribed to the participants in the transcripts to protect privacy. In the transcript extracts provided, the three letter code used in the title is associated with a single institutionalized participant's identity (e.g., WKD indicates a particular institutionalized person with a dementia diagnosis). In the line-by-line extracts, the institutionalized participant is referred to as Mr. or Ms. plus an initial (e.g., Mr. K); the volunteer co-participant is identified using a given name (e.g., Dell).

Investigating Syntactic Patterns Post Dementia Diagnoses

We first present observations from an earlier syntactic analysis derived from twenty conversations with persons diagnosed with dementia (Stickle & Wanner, 2017). Most important to stakeholders who will be conversing with persons diagnosed with dementia is to recognize that they can exhibit syntactic resilience well into the progression of the disease, even under the cognitive pressure of interaction with near strangers. We noted only minor infractions within the execution of verb-argument selection, as well as little evidence of misunderstanding. What this means is that verbs that require a direct object (like *eat*) generally appeared with an appropriate object and that verbs that require a direct and an indirect object (like *give*) generally appeared in the appropriate frame as well.

Additionally, the sentential patterns (i.e., transitivity patterns) selected by persons with dementia paralleled those reported for the general population of English speakers as captured by the *Longman Grammar of Spoken and Written English* (henceforth LGSWE) (Biber et al., 1999).[1] The percentage of non-clausal turns produced by persons diagnosed with dementia, for instance, was in the same range (40.9%) as that found in the Longman conversation corpus (38.6%). In conversations, in general, non-clausal terms are very common.

[1]We chose the LGSWE benchmark corpus to be representative of the syntactic patterns reflective of non-impaired conversational participants as it contains over 3.9 million words in the British English conversation sub-corpus and approximately 2.5 million words in the American English conversation sub-corpus. We compared the LGSWE conversation data to our corpus of 11,482 words obtained from 20 conversations between persons with dementia and their non-impaired co-participants.

For example, a question like "What did you have for breakfast?" is typically not answered with a full clause but rather just a constituent: "Scrambled eggs" (Stickle & Wanner, 2017, Excerpt 2, line 013).

Based on the high percentage of non-clausal units in conversation, Biber et al. (1999, p. 1039) conclude that the sentence as a unit "does not realistically exist in conversational language." They suggest that any meaningful analysis of conversation must take into account situational factors, such as the medium (spoken language cannot be edited and turns therefore are shorter and less elaborate), the discourse situation (face-to-face interaction in a shared space makes the use of syntactic specification and elaboration—for example, through the use of adjectives and adverbs—unnecessary), and the purpose of the conversation (people often share beliefs and opinions, which results in the frequent use of verbs like *think* or *know*). The important point for our purposes here—addressing those who are unfamiliar with seeing transcribed speech—is that during conversation we all speak in ways that if our utterances were transcribed on paper, then they would oftentimes look like fragments and disjointed thought—even for those of us who have no impairment of any kind.

Another area that we noted in which persons with dementia shared speech patterns with non-impaired persons was in their choice of verbs. The most common verbs used by persons with dementia were very similar to those in the LGSWE conversation corpus. They included activity verbs like *come* and *go*, and mental verbs like *know* and *think*, which indicate that speakers in our corpus talked about similar topics as speakers in the LGSWE benchmark corpus. It also should be pointed out that the ten most frequently used verbs that we noted require a variety of syntactic patterns (for example, *come* and *go* are intransitive verbs, while mental verbs like *think* or *know* typically require a subordinate clause to follow), and these requirements were generally met.[2] Three of the most

[2]The most frequently occurring ten verbs in the LGSWE conversation corpus, presented here in descending frequency, are (1) say, (2) **get**, (3) **go**, (4) **know**, (5) **think**, (6) see, (7) **make**, (8) **come**, (9) **take**, and (10) **want** (Biber et al., 1999, p. 375). The most frequently occurring ten verbs in the talk of persons with dementia in our corpus, in descending frequency, are (1) have, (2) **know**, (3) **get**, (4) **come**, (5) **go**, (6) **think**, (7) do, (8) **take**, (9) **want**, (10) **make**/give (Stickle & Wanner, 2017, p. 53). Verbs shared by each are emboldened.

frequent verbs used by both impaired and non-impaired speakers—know, think, want—are verbs that typically require a subordinate clause to follow, in other words, verbs that require complex sentences. In terms of morphological characteristics, such verbs tend to be verbs that have irregular past tense forms (not formed by adding the affix–*ed*), and we did not find any misproductions of these types of verbs.

One interesting difference was that the most frequent verb in the LGSWE corpus, *say*, was not one of the highly used verbs by persons with dementia. This may be related to the fact that patients diagnosed with dementia that reside in a nursing facility have fewer opportunities to participate in conversations and talk about them. (This illustrates the importance of considering context when analyzing conversation.) Another interesting difference between persons with dementia and non-impaired speakers was in regard to verb density: Conversation participants diagnosed with dementia exhibited a higher proportion of verbs in their speech (1 verb per 5.6 words for persons with dementia versus 1 per 10 words for non-impaired). What this means is that when they produced clauses, they used less elaboration in the subject and object phrases than did the non-impaired participants:

"[G]rouper, yes, you eat them" (Stickle & Wanner, 2017, Excerpt 1, line 251).

This suggests that conversation co-participants of persons with dementia should not be surprised if responses sometimes seem even shorter, or more abbreviated, than one is accustomed to in normal conversation.

In general, both the lexical choices and the transitivity patterns paralleled those of the non-impaired participants in the benchmark corpus. It is important to reiterate here, however, that the research just summarized was not investigating in depth the entire range of lexical and syntactic constructions that persons with dementia use in conversation. Our focus was relatively narrow: (1) verbal selection, (2) coordination of verb with correct object selection (transitivity), and (3) proper inflection for tense (morpho-syntactic production). Moreover, the conversations we studied were of "small talk." Given this context, the use of these particular linguistic resources by people with dementia in our study did not look all that different from those found in the speech of unimpaired speakers.

Considering the conversations and use of linguistic resources more broadly, we did, indeed, see linguistic decrement. In terms of interactional facility, however, we found that conversation could proceed even when multiple infractions occurred in the syntactic production of persons diagnosed with dementia. For example, in Extract 1, Ms. Tatter (Ms. T), who has been diagnosed with Alzheimer's disease, displays minor lexical and other types of syntactic difficulties that are hallmark signs of early stages of this progressive disease (American Psychiatric Association, 2013). Ms. Tatter struggles with precise lexical choices, using generic terms instead (i.e., *thing*, *stuff*) (Garcia & Joanette, 1997); she deploys pronouns without sufficient lexical antecedents (e.g., *it*, *them*), and omits noun phrases all together (lines 83, 84) (Hier, Hagenlocker, & Schindler, 1985; Kempler, Andersen, & Henderson, 1995; Ripich & Terrell, 1988). Additionally, Ms. Tatter seems to be having difficulty selecting the correct prepositions (lines 87, 88). We do note that despite relatively felicitous verbal selection, when Ms. Tatter approaches her production of a verb phrase, she produces long pauses (lines 84, 88); cut-offs, i.e., an initial vocalization that stops midstream; and replacements, possible indications of initial difficulty in finding or formulating verb phrases (lines 84–85, 90) (Stickle & Wanner, 2017).[3]

Extract 1: TTR 001 (Stuff inside): Early linguistic decrement

83.	Ms.T:	the thing that I like best of all was uh-
84.		the uh- she ah- (0.7) ra- ah-(1.2)
85.		she rolled the dough out, and
86.	Tom:	Mm
87.	Ms.T:	then she would put ah- this stuff i- in the inside side and (0.5)
88.		and uh- (0.6) put uh- (1.3) I don't know what all she put on

[3]Reports that persons with dementia have difficulty with closed class grammatical items are few. Alegria et al. (2013) showed that preposition use in the talk of persons in moderate stages of Alzheimer's disease were lower than non-impaired persons, but this study concerns comparative usage, not selection error. Meteyard and Patterson (2009) discuss the debate on effects of dementia on closed class retrieval while reporting evidence in their data indicating possible difficulties in preposition selection in the talk of persons diagnosed with semantic dementia.

89.	it,(0.7) but de- then she would roll it out, and (0.7) eh i-
90.	(0.3).h (0.3) we had to- (0.5) pie- - pie tins to uh br- g-
91.	grea:se and she- cut er off and could do it but she had it fixed
92.	to its (1.1) uh- (0.8) degree (0.5) wh- (0.4) that it fit the pan
93.	and when we put them in there they were about that big around and
94.	.h we got them out they were about that big around (0.8)

Despite the length of time and the lack of nouns or verbs that make Ms. Tatter's narrative disjunctive, the co-participant Tom allows Ms. Tatter to tell her narrative without jumping in during the extended pauses. He neither fills in missing words nor reformulates her sentences to make them fit more standard syntax. Instead, he responds with typical receipt tokens (i.e., *mm*, *nice*) (Heritage, 1984, pp. 299–345; Sacks, 1992: II, pp. 521–575; Schegloff, 2007).

Ms. Tatter's linguistic and interactional behaviors appear consistent with the characterization of early to mid-stage Alzheimer's disease causing semantic long-term memory and working memory difficulties that are manifest as trouble producing common words, increased number and length of intra- and inter-turn hesitations, and speech errors (MacDonald, Almor, Henderson, Kempler, & Andersen, 2001). Despite Ms. Tatter's speech errors, she does not display an overt sense that her difficulties could cause problems in the conversation and her co-participant displays no overt signs that these minor disjunctions are actually causing any problems for him. Tom's use of common interlocutor receipt tokens helps keep their conversation flowing.

Thinking Point

Noticing the conversational features emerging within the talk of co-participants diagnosed with dementia may serve to alert caregivers to the many neurological changes that are affecting interactions such as simplified sentence structures, difficulties with word retrieval, possible errors, and increasing signs of frustration due to those changes.

Greater Linguistic Loss and Collaborative Meaning Making

Having presented an extract from a person with dementia in which displays of resilient linguistic, interactional, and pragmatic competency exist despite evidence of lexical and syntactic difficulties, in this next section, we move to participants who appear more obviously impaired. We present extracts in which the talk of participants diagnosed with dementia seems to display greater difficulties with lexical retrieval, memory loss, and difficulty sorting out elements of the past from the present along with greater evidence of syntactic and interactional decrement.

In Extract 2, Ms. Briggs is wandering the common area of her residential facility while engaged in a palilalia loop, the involuntary repetition of one's own speech utterances (Larner, 2015)[4]. The possibility of palilalia (self-repetition) or echolalia (other-repetition) is noted in several neurodegenerative dementias to include Alzheimer's disease (Cruz, 2010), semantic dementia (Kertesz, Jesso, Harciarek, Blair, & McMonagle, 2010), and frontotemporal lobe dementia (Piguet, Hornberger, Shelley, Kipps, & Hodges, 2009). Berthier, Torres-Prioris, and López-Barroso (2017) report that infractions within the bilateral executive-control network[5] that acts as a "brake" preventing inappropriate repetition in healthy brains cannot exert such control and palilalia (or echolalia) may result. For Ms. Briggs (Ms. B), the syntactic loop consists of noun phrases and the past tense "be" verb "was"; however, no complete syntactic–semantic proposition is ever completed during these repetitions.

[4]Also referred to as *recurrent perseveration*, e.g., Bayles, Tomoeda, Kaszniak, Stern, and Eagans (1985).

[5]This area is composed of premotor, posterior parietal and frontal-parietal opercula cortices, right inferior frontal, superior temporal cortices, and basal ganglia.

Extract 2: BGG 002a (The Kathy): Palilalia looping

16.	Ms. B:	the Kathy, the Kathy, was Kathy, was Kathy, that was Kathy,
17.		and that was Kathy, so, have we, and Kathy, and the Kathy
18.		and the Kathy and the Kathy, and the Kathy. but, that
19.		was the Kathy, the Kathy, the Kathy, the Kathy, the Kathy,

As Ms. Briggs nears the student volunteer Tom and his conversation partner Robert, something remarkable occurs as Tom begins to interact with her: the palilalia loop is broken and Ms. Briggs competently engages in conversation. Hearing Ms. Brigg's palilalia utterance, Tom treats it as both having sufficient syntax and doing the work (i.e., action) of a question. Specifically, Tom responds as if Ms. Briggs is inquiring the whereabouts of "Kathy" (line 20). After nine-tenths of a second, Ms. Briggs provides an appropriate response to Tom's answer to her presumed question (lines 22–25).

Extract 3: BGG 002b (I hadn't seen Kathy): Breaking the palilalia loop

19.	MS. B:	[The Kathy, the Kathy,]
20.	Tom:	[I hadn't seen Kathy.]
21.		(0.9)
22.	MS. B:	okay.
23.		(0.4)
24.	MS. B:	which mean- they're ou see, they're ru- they're really,
25.		really ni-, they're night, outta, outta here.
26.	Tom:	oh yeah.
27.	MS. B:	okay?
28.	Tom:	Okay. .hh
29	MS. B:	is there anything else, anything else there is?
30		(0.4)
31	Tom:	ha(ah)-I, I think we're all set(h).
32.	Ms. B:	Okay=

While her syntax still displays some disjointedness, she indicates that since Tom has not seen Kathy, Kathy must not be here, and states that she (or they) is "outta here," perhaps signifying that it is nighttime (lines

24–25). Here, we conjecture, that Ms. Briggs' involuntary defective syntactic loop is interrupted and, through Tom's utterance, a consequential, subsequent syntactic (and fitted semantic) process is put into play. This new and competent syntactic chain is primed by Tom's "answer." Ms. Briggs is, then, able to engage in a linguistic processing plan fitted to her interlocutor.

At line 29, Ms. Briggs initiates a turn of talk that displays a role reversal which is fitted to continuing conversation. Rather than being the recipient of help, she asks a question as helper: "is there anything else, anything else there is?." Note that her first utterance displays adherence to standard syntax and is complete, while her second utterance topicalizes the subject complement "anything else," placing it in first position in the utterance. (This could signal the beginning of another palilalia loop, but one does not occur at this time.) With Tom's response (line 31), he indicates both surprise at Ms. Briggs' polite request to ensure he and Robert, "her guests," have what they need. Tom closes this sequence by confirming that he and Robert do, indeed, have what they need, signifying nothing is required of Ms. Briggs (line 31). As Ms. Briggs acknowledges Tom's response with an "okay" (line 32), Tom continues to engage her by bringing her into the existing conversation with Mr. Thurman (i.e., Robert). This engagement affords Ms. Briggs a window for additional conversation that is produced with sufficient syntax, even if it does not adhere to Standard English (see Extract 4).

Extract 4: BGG 002c (Do you know Robert): The dignity of conversation

33.	Tom:	=do you know, do you know R↑obert?
34.		(0.4)
35.	Ms. B:	yeah.
36.		(0.3)

Both Ms. Briggs and Tom produce recognizable closing actions as shown in Extract 5 (lines 38–48). As the conversation ends, Ms. Briggs' voice is heard on the audio to reduce in volume, indicative of her turning and walking away from the recording device, and her palilalia talk returns (lines 49–51).

Extract 5: BGG 002c: (Have a good day): Closing the conversation

37.	Tom:	ye[ah.]
38.	Ms. B:	[yeah. and, I didn't, I think that was, I think that was all
39.		I'll, I'll uh, uh, that was all all I'll dis- cuss it again.
40.		yeah. o[kay.]
41.	Tom:	[okay.]
42.		(0.3)
43.	Tom:	well, I'll let you know if I see her.
44.		(0.3)
45.	Ms. B:	okay.
46.		(0.5)
47.	Ms. B:	ha(h) O(h)k[(ha)ay.
48.	Tom:	[hav(ha)have] have a good day..hh
49.	Ms. B:	ok(h)ay. y(h)ou t(h)wo do the sa- I (know) ya can't- and I say
50.		oh, my golly, I know I hope, I hope I don't get Kathy, I
51.		mean Kathy, Kathy, Kathy.

This extract is but one instance of a co-participant treating a dementia resident's palilalia loop as meaningful, thus resulting in successful interaction, that is, genuine conversation. It is as if Tom's "answer" to Ms. Brigg's "question" derails the singular-tracked, uncontrollable, repetitive monologue and initiates a different linguistic pathway, one that is suited for—primed and coordinated—dialogue and interaction. From this single instance, we foresee this phenomenon as a potential practice; it may be one way to achieve engagement with folks who suffer from these linguistic effects due to neurocognitive insult. This and similar co-participant strategies could, potentially, serve research agendas to help persons with dementia experience increased interaction, engagement, and, possibly, prolonged linguistic competence.

Thinking Point

Treating a co-participant's talk as meaningful despite displays of conversational difficulties may allow a window for more accurate production—structural, semantic, and pragmatic actions—and better ensure all co-participants experience dignity during the interaction.

Language, Communication, and Personhood Loss: Co-participant Strategies

In the following extended extract, Mr. Thatcher is shown as having difficulty producing the necessary lexical and syntactic constructions to consistently assemble contextually meaningful utterances. He also displays an awareness of these difficulties (Ripich, Vertes, Whitehouse, Fulton, & Ekelman, 1991) and their potential interactional problems, an awareness that has been observed in the design of turns of persons well into the later stages of Alzheimer's disease (Müller & Guendouzi, 2005). Mr. Thatcher's repeated use of *I don't know* utterances in concert with exacerbations and response cries (Goffman, 1981) can be heard as an extended complaint sequence or, what may be more specifically described as an exposition on loss, both language and identity. We present this case to illustrate how a person with dementia instantiates these losses through limited syntax and incredible disruptions in lexical retrieval, common aspects of late-stage dementia, before we then examine co-participant strategies that work to initiate a coordinated dialogue which, ultimately, lead to a more engaged, coherent conversation.

We begin with Mr. Thatcher's launch of an extended complaint sequence. His multiunit turn of talk reveals extensive linguistic loss during this period of the conversation, as captured in the transcript details. We see evidence of extreme agrammatism; effortful, halting speech with inconsistent speech sound errors; and apraxia of speech (distortions) in syntax, phonology, and semantics. This cluster of deficits is most associated with progressive non-fluent aphasia (PNFA) (Gorno-Tempini et al., 2011) that arises from atrophy in the left inferior frontal cortex, anterior insula, dorsolateral prefrontal cortex, and superior temporal cortex (Peelle & Grossman, 2008).

The extract begins as Mr. Thatcher (Mr. T) launches a complaint about someone having left a door open, making the entrance vulnerable to whomever should want in (lines 42–43). We highlight Mr. Thatcher's difficulty in selecting contextually appropriate lexical and syntactic resources.

Extract 6: THW 001a (They give you a diamond): Impaired syntax

42.	Mr. T:	they don't do anything about (.)
43.		what they do wi- d- with- (.)
44.		the door that you would open to whoever ah wants.
45.		well, that's bad.
46.	Jim:	yeah, it [is.]
47.	Mr. T:	[Um,]
48.		(1.8)
49.	Mr. T:	when you get over there-
50.		(1.5)
51.	Mr. T:	they give you a (diamond).
52.		(0.9)
53.	Jim:	yeah.
54.	Mr. T:	Ish-
55.		(2.3)
56.	Mr. T:	are ya'll fixing to do it?
57.	Jim:	yeah.
58.		(6.7)
59.	Jim:	they might.
60.		(45.0)
61.	Jim:	well, the lunch looks good.
62.		(0.4)
63.	Jim:	we should go have some of your lunch.
64.		(11.1)

While some of Mr. Thatcher's talk is understandable despite lexical and syntactic difficulties (lines 42–45), other utterances appear out of context and indecipherable (lines 47–51). Jim, the student volunteer, provides minimal response tokens common to active engagement during mundane conversations (lines 46, 53, 57, 59). Jim then makes a suggestion that the two get some lunch (line 63). Mr. Thatcher, however, does not address Jim's suggestion and, instead, continues with more self-focused talk revealing an awareness of his losses.

Extract 7: THW 001b (Haven't got a clue): Recognition

65.	Mr. T:	that makes-
66.		(1.5)
67.	Mr. T:	~N~O:
68.		(5.9)

69.	Mr. T:	(woosey/moosey.)
70.		(11.7)
71.	Jim:	u'huh.
72.		(71.6)
73.	Mr. T:	I don't know.
74.		(0.8)
75.	Mr. T:	I haven't got a clue.
76.		(1.6)
77.	Jim:	Yeah.

Not addressing Jim's lunch suggestion, Mr. Thatcher begins a new topic. After difficulty producing a syntactically or semantically coherent utterance, in line 73, Mr. Thatcher produces an appropriate and syntactically complete "I don't know." This utterance is followed by the formulaic phrase "I haven't got a clue" (line 75) which reiterates an awareness of his inabilities. Jim continues providing minimal response tokens that seem to encourage Mr. Thatcher's continued talk (lines 71, 77).

Being an Empathetic Recipient

As Mr. Thatcher continues, his talk becomes more poignant, addressing his losses.

Extract 8: THW 001d (What to ask): A window into loss

189.	Mr. T:	no, I don't (.) ha:ve any,
190.		(0.8)
191.	Mr. T:	more-
192.		(1.9)
193.		have ah-
194.		(1.0)
195.	Jim:	yeah.
196.		[(9.4)
197.		[((crying))]
198.	Jim:	mm.
199.		(1.5)
200.	Jim:	I know it's hard.
201.		(2.9)
202.	Jim:	It's difficult.
203.		(113.7)

204.	Jim:	yeah.
205.		(2.1)
206.	Mr. T:	I don't know where to go.
207.		(0.5)
208.	Mr. T:	I don't know what s'to go.
209.		(0.3)
210.	Mr. T:	I don't know what to a:sk.
211.		(0.6)
212.	Jim:	yeah.

Despite the gaps within Mr. Thatcher's utterances, the disruptions in his syntax and lexical retrieval, and his affective response of crying, Jim allows his co-participant to continue talking. He does not attempt to assuage Mr. Thatcher's emotional state or offer any "bright side" comments. He does not offer syntactic or lexical corrections. Instead, he provides minimal receipt tokens (lines 195, 198, 212); the interactional space to finish his utterances; and expressions of empathy: "I know it's hard" (line 200) and "It's difficult" (line 202). In short, Jim defers control of the interaction to Mr. Thatcher and provides overt signs of both engaged listening and understanding.

During the next twelve minutes of conversation, Mr. Thatcher's talk continues to fluctuate from indecipherable to moments of relative coherence. He seems to show an understanding of the recorder: "I know what this thing is doing. (2.0) That box" (lines 247–249, not shown). He complains about his family (or someone) putting down his dog: "Some of them put 'em do:wn. (0.5) What- they p- put down for (.) my dog" (lines 265–267, not shown). He continues to display dissatisfaction about his life and expresses that he wishes to be normal again (line 295, not shown). Yet, despite the incredible linguistic and interactional problems displayed in Mr. Thatcher's talk, toward the end of the conversation, he is able to turn the focus of his talk away from self and toward Jim.

Restoring Self and Sense to the Interaction

Mr. Thatcher turns the topic of talk to Jim's life. The talk still exhibits linguistic and interactional difficulty but shows greater syntactic and semantic facility than his earlier talk.

Extract 9: THW 001e (Where 'bouts are you): A moment's control

300.	Mr. T:	Where bouts are you?
301.		(2.1)
302.	Jim:	Me?
303.		(0.4)
304.	Mr. T:	yeah.
305.	Jim:	I'm in, uh,
306.		(0.7)
307.	Jim:	Charlotte.
308.		(1.4)
309.	Jim:	I live over near the university?
310.		(6.3)
311.	Mr. T:	yeah.
312.		(1.0)

While Jim seems taken aback at the (now) relative competence of Mr. Thatcher's question (line 300), as evidenced by his response "Me?" uttered with a questioning intonation (line 302), he assumes the role of interviewee, matching his own tempo with that of his co-participant. As the conversation draws to its close, Mr. Thatcher continues to exert a more collaborative role, coordinating his discourse to better fit his interlocutor and, simultaneously, his command over syntactic, lexical, and semantic fluency is increased.

Extract 10: THW 001f (Answers I got): Collaborative conversation

313.	Mr. T:	you betchu want answers I got?
314.		(1.0)
315.	Jim:	yeah.
316.		(1.0)
317.	Mr. T:	the only one.
318.	Jim:	it's a good answer.
319.		(22.0)

```
320. Jim:     hmm.
321.          (20.6)
322. Mr. T:   the only thing I can think of,
323.          (0.9)
324. Jim:     yeah. ((sniff)) ma(h)n.
```
End of transcript

Mr. Thatcher's utterance at line 313 shows an awareness that Jim's task is to retrieve answers (perhaps because he has seen Jim's audio recorder). His linguistic formulation is both better fitted and better formed. Mr. Thatcher states he has, at least, one answer (line 317), the only thing he can think of (line 322). Here, Mr. Thatcher displays an epistemic stance with a positive tilt, in contrast to his earlier multiple claims of insufficient knowledge, the inability to say anything, and uncertainty. As the talk develops, Jim displays to Mr. Thatcher (and us) that he has come to some understanding of Mr. Thatcher's experience living with dementia ("I know it's hard," line 200). The strategies employed by Jim keep Mr. Thatcher engaged in ways that seemingly lead to the retrieval of better fitted linguistic resources. These strategies include sufficient wait time during long pauses which allows his co-participant with dementia the needed warm up period (Stickle & Wanner, 2017) to express whatever is necessary and however possible. Jim also displays empathy. Jim's use of minimal receipt tokens—not corrections or palliative responses—are indicative of active listening while his utterances serve to prime Mr. T's utterances and restore a sense of interactional competence to his co-participant by allowing coordination between the two interlocutors. We conjecture that it may be these kinds of co-participant strategies that allow for increased and prolonged interactions with persons diagnosed with dementia, even at later stages.

Thinking Points

Despite increasing linguistic, interactional, and personhood loss, co-participants might help trigger restored interactional competency to persons diagnosed with dementia by deferring control, exhibiting overt signs of engaged listening, and displaying empathy.

Summary

We looked at three cases. In the first, the individual with dementia exhibited linguistic and interactional skills with minimal syntactic errors with no evidence within the conversation, from either participant, of interactional trouble resulting. This level of ability is not uncommon in persons with early to mid-stage dementia (American Psychiatric Association, 2013). Consequently, in this case, conversation proceeded in fairly normal ways. In the other two cases, by contrast, we looked at persons who exhibited more severe linguistic decrement characteristic of late-stage illness (e.g., palilalia; utterances with ill-formed syntax; American Psychiatric Association, 2013). Trouble often arose in the conversations. The persons with dementia would utter statements that were not comprehensible, thus making it unclear how a co-participant should proceed. Despite these difficulties the persons with dementia could, on occasion, use language that was more syntactically well-formed and better fitted to the conversation.

Our analysis suggests that treating co-participants' incoherent or otherwise ill-formed talk as though it were sensible may have facilitated these occasional moments of relatively well-formed syntax and interaction. Tom, for example, treats Ms. B's palilalia loop "the Kathy, the Kathy, the Kathy …" as *though* Ms. B is asking of the whereabouts of Kathy. In other words, he treats her utterances as though they were a sensible attempt at asking a question. Jim, on the other hand, gives Mr. T plenty of interactional space (i.e., time) and liberty (i.e., freedom from correction—factual or linguistic) to allow him to say what he is able to say. This suggests the need for a warm up period for the person with dementia (Stickle & Wanner, 2017).[6] We consider our findings to support the importance of syntactic priming (Bock, 1986, 1990; Pickering & Branigan, 1998) and evidence of syntactic coordination in

[6]This evidence supports the view that syntactic evidence is housed in the lemma stratum (Pickering & Branigan, 1998; Roelofs, 1992) and the psycholinguistic model positing that language production relies on a three stage process: (1) a prelinguistic phase, (2) a phase of linguistic formulation that is aligned with and fitted to the intended interlocutor prior to linguistic expression, and (3) linguistic expression (Dell, 1986; Levelt, 1989; Levelt, Roelofs, & Meyer, 1999).

dialogue (Branigan, Pickering, McLean, & Cleland, 2007). Awareness of these connections may help guide participants in their selections of topics, language used, and tempo of the talk when conversing with persons with dementia.

Further helpful strategies might include supplying appropriate interactional cues that demonstrate active listening and, when appropriate, empathy. Lastly, yielding control of the conversation to the person with dementia can initiate more fitted linguistic resources and increase levels of engagement allowing for longer, more productive interactions. These strategies appear to instantiate dignity and competence to persons with compromised linguistic faculties allowing conversations to be truly collaborative events.

While we recognize these last two Alzheimer's case studies are just that—two cases—we are hopeful that the co-participant strategies noted here are applicable in other situations as we have drawn attention to those linguistic and interactional behaviors that are also symptomatic of other types of dementias. Knowing what linguistic and interactional resources persons with dementia have available during actual conversations, which ones they are more (or less) likely to use in mundane conversation, and how, specifically, these resources can be engaged by the practices employed by their co-participants helps lay a firm foundation on which to build additional studies with a more applied focus and, ultimately, contributes to best communication practices for family, caregivers, and practitioners use.

Practical Highlights

1. Treating the talk of persons diagnosed with dementia as meaningful actions may help restore a sense of identity and allow a window for better communication.
2. Yielding control of the conversation to persons diagnosed with dementia may result in their increased ability to access syntactic and lexical structures.
3. Displaying empathy rather than sympathy may encourage persons with dementia to engage, rather than withdraw, during interaction.

References

Alegria, R., Gallo, C., Bolso, M., dos Santos, B., Prisco, C. R., Bottino, C., & Ines, N. M. (2013). Comparative study of the uses of grammatical categories: Adjectives, adverbs, pronouns, interjections, conjunctions and prepositions in patients with Alzheimer's disease. *Alzheimer's & Dementia: The Journal of the Alzheimer's Association, 9*(4), P882.

American Psychiatric Association. (2013). *Neurocognitive disorders.* In *Diagnostic and statistical manual of mental disorders* (5th ed.). Washington, DC: n.a. http://dx.doi.org/10.1176/appi.books.9780890425596.neurocognitivedisorders.

Atkinson, J. M., & Heritage, J. (Eds.). (1984). *Structures of social action.* Cambridge, UK: Cambridge University Press.

Bayles, K. A., Tomoeda, C. K., Kaszniak, A. W., Stern, L. Z., & Eagans, K. K. (1985). Verbal perseveration of dementia patients. *Brain and Language, 25,* 102–116.

Berthier, M. L., Torres-Prioris, M. J., & López-Barroso, D. (2017). Thinking on treating echolalia in aphasia: Recommendations and caveats for future research directions. *Frontiers in Human Neuroscience, 11,* https://doi.org/10.3389/fnhum.2017.00164.

Biber, D., Johansson, S., Leech, G., Conrad, S., Finegan, E., & Quirk, R. (1999). *Longman grammar of spoken and written English* (Vol. 2). Cambridge, MA: MIT Press.

Bock, K. (1986). Syntactic persistence in language production. *Cognitive Psychology, 18,* 355–387.

Bock, K. (1990). Structure in language: Creating form in talk. *American Psychologist, 45*(11), 1221–1236. https://doi.org/10.1037/0003-066X.45.11.1221.

Branigan, H. P., Pickering, M. J., McLean, J. F., & Cleland, A. A. (2007). Syntactic alignment and participant role in dialogue. *Cognition, 104*(2), 163–197.

Cruz, F. M. D. (2010). Verbal repetitions and palilalia in Alzheimer's discourse. *Clinical Linguistics & Phonetics, 24*(11), 848–858.

Dell, G. S. (1986). A spreading-activation theory of retrieval in sentence production. *Psychological Review, 93*(3), 283–321.

Garcia, L. J., & Joanette, Y. (1997). Analysis of conversational topic shifts: A multiple case study. *Brain and Language, 58,* 92–114.

Goffman, E. (1981). *Forms of talk.* Philadelphia: University of Pennsylvania Press.

Gorno-Tempini, M. L., Hillis, A. E., Weintraub, S., Kertesz, A., Mendez, M., Cappa, S. E. E. A., ... Manes, F. (2011). Classification of primary progressive aphasia and its variants. *Neurology, 76*(11), 1006–1014.

Heritage, J. (1984). A change-of-state token and aspects of its sequential placement. In J. M. Atkinson & J. Heritage (Eds.), *Structures of social action: Studies in conversation analysis* (pp. 299–345). New York, NY: Cambridge University Press.

Hier, D. B., Hagenlocker, D., & Schindler, A. G. (1985). Language disintegration in dementia: Effects of etiology and severity. *Brain and Language, 25,* 117–133.

Jefferson, G. (2004). Glossary of transcript symbols with an introduction. *Pragmatics and Beyond New Series, 125,* 13–34.

Kempler, D., Andersen, E. S., & Henderson, V. W. (1995). Linguistic and attentional contributions to anomia in Alzheimer's disease: A comparison of off-line vs. on-line sentence processing. *Neuropsychiatry, Neuropsychology, and Behavioral Neurology, 8,* 33–37.

Kertesz, A., Jesso, S., Harciarek, M., Blair, M., & McMonagle, P. (2010). What is semantic dementia? A cohort study of diagnostic features and clinical boundaries. *Archives of Neurology, 67,* 483–489. https://doi.org/10.1001/archneurol.2010.55.

Larner, A. J. (2015, July–August). Neurological signs: Echo phenomena. *ACNR, 15*(3), 16.

Levelt, W. I. M. (1989). *Speaking: From intention to articulation.* Cambridge, MA: MIT Press.

Levelt, W. J., Roelofs, A., & Meyer, A. S. (1999). A theory of lexical access in speech production. *Behavioral and Brain Sciences, 22*(1), 1–38.

MacDonald, M. C., Almor, A., Henderson, V. W., Kempler, D., & Andersen, E. S. (2001). Assessing working memory and language comprehension in Alzheimer's disease. *Brain and Language, 78*(1), 17–42.

Meteyard, L., & Patterson, K. (2009). The relation between content and structure in language production: An analysis of speech errors in semantic dementia. *Brain and Language, 110*(3), 121–134.

Müller, N., & Guendouzi, J. A. (2005). Order and disorder in conversation: Encounters with dementia of the Alzheimer's type. *Clinical Linguistics & Phonetics, 19*(5), 393–404.

Peelle, J. E., & Grossman, M. (2008). Language processing in frontotemporal dementia: A brief review. *Language and Linguistics Compass, 2*(1), 18–35.

Pickering, M. J., & Branigan, H. P. (1998). The representation of verbs: Evidence from syntactic priming in language production. *Journal of Memory and Language, 39*(4), 633–651.
Piguet, O., Hornberger, M., Shelley, B. P., Kipps, C. M., & Hodges, J. R. (2009). Sensitivity of current criteria for the diagnosis of behavioral variant frontotemporal dementia. *Neurology, 72,* 732–737.
Pope, C., & Davis, B. H. (2011). Finding a balance: The Carolinas Conversation Collection. *Corpus Linguistics and Linguistic Theory, 7*(1), 143–161.
Ripich, D. N., Vertes, D., Whitehouse, P., Fulton, S., & Ekelman, B. (1991). Turn-taking and speech act patterns in the discourse of senile dementia of the Alzheimer's type patients. *Brain and Language, 40*(3), 330–343.
Ripich, D. N., & Terrell, B. Y. (1988). Patterns of discourse cohesion and coherence in Alzheimer's disease. *Journal of Speech and Hearing Disorders, 53,* 8–15.
Roelofs, A. (1992). A spreading-activation theory of lemma retrieval in speaking. *Cognition, 42*(1–3), 107–142.
Ryan, E. B., Bannister, K. A., & Anas, A. P. (2009). The dementia narrative: Writing to reclaim social identity. *Journal of Aging Studies, 23*(3), 145–157.
Sacks, H. (1992). *Lectures on conversation* (2 Vols.; Fall 1964–Spring 1972). Oxford, UK: Blackwell.
Schegloff, E. A. (2007). *Sequence organization in interaction: A primer in conversation analysis.* Cambridge, UK: Cambridge University Press.
Stickle, T., & Wanner, A. (2017). Transitivity patterns exhibited by persons with dementia in conversation. *Applied Linguistics, 40*(1), 43–63.

Recommended Readings

Foundational Studies

Davis, B. H. (Ed.). (2005). *Alzheimer talk, text and context: Enhancing communication.* New York, NY: Palgrave Macmillan.
Guendouzi, J., & Muller, N. (2006). *Approaches to discourse in dementia.* Mahwah, NJ: Erlbaum.
Hamilton, H. E. (2005). *Conversations with an Alzheimer's patient: An interactional sociolinguistic study.* Cambridge, UK: Cambridge University Press.

Ramanathan, V. (1997). *Alzheimer discourse: Some sociolinguistic dimensions.* Mahwah, NJ: Erlbaum.

Sabat, S. R. (2001). *The experience of Alzheimer's disease: Life through a tangled veil.* Oxford, UK: Blackwell.

Emerging Research

Banovic, S., Zunic, L. J., & Sinanovic, O. (2018). Communication difficulties as a result of dementia. *Materia Socio-Medica, 30*(3), 221–224.

Davis, B. H., & Maclagan, M. (2018). Narrative and ageing: Exploring the range of narrative types in dementia conversation. *European Journal of English Studies, 22*(1), 76–90.

Leiros, B. G., Méndez, L. P., Huerta, M. Z., Eguinoa, L. M., García-Bragado, F., Alvarez, T. T., & Larreta, J. R. (2018). Prevalence and concordance between the clinical and the post-mortem diagnosis of dementia in a psychogeriatric clinic. *Neurología* (English Edition), *33*(1), 13–17.

McGilton, K. S., Rochon, E., Sidani, S., Shaw, A., Ben-David, B. M., Saragosa, M., ... Pichora-Fuller, M. K. (2017). Can we help care providers communicate more effectively with persons having dementia living in long-term care homes? *American Journal of Alzheimer's Disease & Other Dementias*, *32*(1), 41–50.

7

Foregrounding Competence in Interaction with a Person with Dementia: Co-participant Responses to Disordered Talk

Lyndsay Lindley

Learning Objectives

By the end of this chapter, you will be able to:

- Discuss different strategies for responding to disordered or confused talk;
- Recognize evidence of retained interactional competence in persons with dementia;
- Better employ strategies to use within interactions with persons with dementia, particularly ones that help facilitate and validate personhood.

L. Lindley (✉)
Department of Social Policy and Social Work,
University of York, York, UK
e-mail: lyndsay.lindley@york.ac.uk

T. Stickle (ed.), *Learning from the Talk of Persons with Dementia*,
The Language of Mental Health, https://doi.org/10.1007/978-3-030-43977-4_7

Introduction

Despite difficulties incurred when researching the lives and language of persons with dementia,[1] this chapter demonstrates the ecological richness that can be gleaned from careful analysis of quotidian interactions between persons with dementia and their daily co-participants within a range of naturally occurring contexts. Aligning with new research motives that highlight ways in which abilities, independence, and quality of life are maintained (Mok & Müller, 2014; Quince, 2011; Sabat & Lee, 2011), this chapter,[2] focuses on the interactional competence of a person with dementia and reveals ways in which her independence is facilitated and her personhood validated by her interlocutors. As such, this chapter demonstrates ways that co-participants can respond to disordered talk in order that family members, carers, clinicians, and researchers may informedly choose their own resources in the hope of facilitating better conversations with persons diagnosed with dementia for all participants involved.

Data

Two focal participants who initially agreed to take part were a woman, referred to as "Dana," who was 88 years of age, living in her own home seven years after a dementia diagnosis, and her primary caregiver, her son, referred to as "John." Following the initial meeting with the dyad, further conversational participants from the family and community agreed to take part. All were consented and ascribed pseudonyms to protect their identities (Table 7.1).

The aim of the data collection was to obtain, as near possible, natural conversations. Participants were trained to use a small, portable recording device so that they could record any part of their daily life and interactions. Constant dialogue was not necessary and no special activities or topics

---

[1] E.g., ethically obtaining data and informed consent, collecting data under artificial or forced contexts, poorly developed relationships between researcher and person with dementia, time and stress constraints asked of caregivers who must participate, as well as a host of others.

[2] Note: This study is a subpart of a wider study on family interaction (Lindley, 2016).

Table 7.1 Participants' demographic information

Participant pseudonym	Age	Relationship to person with dementia (Dana)	Role	Ethnographic interview
Dana	88		Person with dementia	
John	61	Son	Primary Caregiver	Yes
Maureen	59	Daughter-in-law	Caregiver	Yes
Emma	33	Granddaughter		
Mick	51		Visiting chiropodist	
Hal	–		Hairdresser	
George	50	Son	Caregiver	
Trudy	–	Daughter-in-law	Caregiver	
Chloe	15	Granddaughter		
Barney	13	Grandson		

Source Author

were required. This allowed the participants to record as they wished. From November 2012 to January 2013, a total of 15 hours of audio data were recorded. The full corpus of recordings included mealtimes, watching television, car journeys, a visit from the chiropodist, and a recording of one of Dana's weekly appointments at her hairdresser's salon.

Methods

The corpus of 15 hours of conversation is explored primarily through applied conversation analysis. Conversation analysis, as noted previously in this volume, consists of a close, turn-by-turn analysis of talk which aims to show how co-participants collaboratively make meaning and complete actions.

Additionally, ethnographic methods were used: an interview was conducted, jointly, with Dana's two primary caregivers which took place after all audio data had been collected in order that fact-checking could be carried out with reference to the conversational data, for example, Dana's life history (see Extract 1) and diagnosis. The semi-structured interview took one hour, forty minutes and was primarily participant-led, exploring the experience of the caregivers. Further, observational data were collected at the weekly singing group that Dana attended. Permission was given by the Alzheimer's Society to participate and observe at the group.

Overview

The practices of Dana's co-participants in responding to episodes of disorder and confusion fall into three general categories[3]:

1. Alignment with the disordered or confused talk through
   a. minimal tokens
   b. generalized response
   c. collusion
2. Repair initiation (i.e., cues to correct) by
   a. significant delay, or no response
   b. other means
3. Correction of errant talk

Interlocutor Responses to Disordered Talk: Alignment

Minimal Response

When co-participants make the choice not to correct errant talk they may produce a next turn in the form of a minimal token (e.g., *right, yeah, unhuh, okay*). Illustrating this practice, Extract 1 is a conversation between Dana and her thirteen-year-old grandson, Barney. They have been talking about school and Barney has asked Dana where she went to school. We pick up the conversation as Dana answers this.

---

[3]The range of possible responses observed here is similar to that noted by Lindholm (2015). In her study of responses to confabulation, Lindholm found practices ranged on a continuum from noncommitment to acquiescence.

Extract 1: LML7-4.14930

01.	Dana:	oh I was born an reared in Belfast ah had all mi
02.		children in Belfast
03.	Barney:	£uhh ri(h)ght£.
04.	Dana:	Yea
05.		(0.5)
06.	Dana:	and your dad
07.	Barney:	yeah.

Dana is confabulating about the birthplace of her children when she states that all her children were born in Belfast, Northern Ireland, and specifies (line 6) "and your dad," referencing Barney's father. Her sons, in fact, were born in the North of England, Barney's dad being the youngest. Barney does not correct or query Dana's statement in any way but, instead, responds with minimal tokens *right* and *yeah*, aligning with Dana's story. Relational constraints do, of course, exist on these interlocutors: is it appropriate, in such conversations, for a thirteen-year-old boy to correct his grandmother? (Wardaugh & Fuller, 2015). Nonetheless, the machinery is available to him if he were to pursue the spurious fact, and he chooses not to do so.

Generalized Response

A further example of an aligning turn which does not attempt a repair initiation is a generalized response (e.g., formulaic responses, generic comments). In Extract 2, Dana is talking about her late husband in the present tense.

Extract 2: LML1-9.1656

01.	Dana:	your dad has no trouble with sleeping
02.		(.)
03.	John:	Hum
04.	Dana:	he'd sleep from now to doomsday
05.		(0.4)
06.	Dana:	hehe hehehu °hahaha° hohoho hehe god help'm
07.		(5.6)

08.	Dana:	he would
09.		(1.8)
10.	Dana:	if he could but
11.		[he can't]
12.	Mauree:	[there's lots] of people like that
13.	Dana:	yea huhu

Dana mentions her late husband, referring to him in the present tense in line 1, a practice that occurs many times in the data. Note that John aligns with the turn in line 3 with a minimal token and passes up the opportunity to repair or correct Dana's statement. Lines 8–11 are built as a formulaic phrase: "he would if he could but he can't" and it is ambiguous whether Dana is continuing to speak about her husband in the present or whether she has recognized that he is no longer living.

In line 12, Maureen responds to Dana with a generalized, aligning turn. Maureen's turn is not constructed with Dana's husband as the subject, but, rather, she employs the general subject "lots of people like that." Potter (1996, p. 168) states that "vague propositions" and "broad categorizations" are robust in conversation since they are not attached to individual perceptions or emotions and are not easily contradicted. Potter's observation is inverted in this example in that the generalization allows Maureen to align with the disordered talk without contradicting Dana's perception of reality. By adopting this practice, Maureen sustains the social interaction and avoids any potential upset which might occur by reminding Dana that her husband is dead. This also avoids the dilemma of whether to collude with the delusional state of the person with dementia, which many caregivers struggle with and see as deceitful (Blum, 1994; Day, James, Meyer, & Lee, 2011; Tuckett, 2012).

Colluding Response

The third practice of aligning with the disordered talk is to collude with the perceived reality of the person with dementia. By doing this, co-participants explicitly take a stance that is contrary to what they know to be real or true so that their stance aligns with the interlocutor. This is similar to Lindholm's (2015, p. 194) categorization of "elaborate confirming responses" to confabulation in which the interlocutor explicitly aligns with a view they know not to be true. This chapter does not consider the ethics of such practices but, rather, considers only the interactional outcomes of various responses to delusion.

Examining colluding responses in Extracts 3 and 4, below, the problematic outcome of John's colluding in Dana's delusion relating to the family photograph becomes evident.

Extract 3: LML1-11.2980

01.	John:	NO YE CAN'T HAVE ANY'am afraid
02.	Dana:	no'am not taking it down no
03.	John:	tell'em! tell'em they can't have any
04.	Dana:	no don't tell them anything! (.)they're in
05.		picture an' they're staying there
06.	John:	oh right

In lines 1–3, John has joined in with Dana by treating the people in the photograph as real, alive, present. In lines 4–5, unexpectedly, Dana contradicts her son, recognizing for herself the delusion in their joint talk. She introduces reality: "they're in the picture an' they're staying there." John's falsity is brought to light, and he must change his stance by aligning with his mother's new found clarity. Moments later, however, Dana returns to the delusion that the people in the photograph are real, alive, present (see Extract 4):

Extract 4: LML1-11.3011

01.	Dana	hh so. are you gonna eat your tea with thim
02.	John:	with you
03.	Dana:	at the table
04.	John:	with <u>you</u>!
05.	Dana:	b-y-bd=↑what↑ about them two
06.		(3.2)
07.	Dana:	you're not gonna give them anything=
08.	John:	=↑no↑: it's [justaf:
09.	Dana:	[thi gonna]hang on the wall
10.	John:	shjust a ↑pho:↑tograph
11.	Dana:	ha:hahahaha[ha ha ha
12.	John:	[£they can't] come down and ea:t£

13.	Dana:	hu ha ha ↑ho:::↑ hhmm hm ↑hm hm↑
14.		(0.3)
15.	Dana:	hhh £they can't come down and eat£
16.	John:	no:
17.	Dana:	£I'll jump on ih£ (.)
18.		£I'll take it down and jump on it .hh an'
19.		you'll have your m:other, your sisters, your
20.		brother, and all of them£=

When Dana returns to the delusion (Extract 4, line 5), John finds himself sticking to reality, telling his mother the vision is "just a photograph" (line 10). John's assertion of reality does not, however, break Dana's delusion (lines 17–20).

Colluding with disorder is a very rare practice in these data. Extracts 3 and 4 demonstrate the interactional problems that interlocutors face when a person with dementia's perception of reality fluctuates. Co-participants' deception can be exposed, and they may find themselves "stranded" in a disordered reality. On the other hand, attempting to bring the person with dementia back to reality has its own challenges which may include failure (as seen above) or, even, argument and stress (which will be discussed in the section "Corrections").

Thinking Points

- Neither minimal nor generalized responses to delusional/nonfactual talk appear to cause interactional difficulties.
- Colluding responses to delusional/nonfactual talk also do not seem to cause interactional difficulties.
- This remains true even if the person with dementia gains clarity during the interaction and self corrects; such moments may allow the person with dementia the ability to take control of any necessary correction.
- Overall, the use of minimal, generalized, and colluding responses could prove helpful to sustaining interaction.

Interlocutor Responses to Disordered Talk: Delays and Repair Initiation

As documented in other conversation analytic investigations of communication disorders (inter alia Hamilton, 1994; Perkins, Whitworth, & Lesser, 1998; Müller & Guendouzi, 2005; Guendouzi & Müller, 2006; Mikesell, 2009), people with dementia retain the ability to initiate repair on their own and others' talk. Even in the later stages of dementia, when verbal skills are severely impaired, Hamilton (1994, p. 61) showed that a person with dementia can initiate other-repair through the use of intonation and non-lexical utterances such as *huh* or *hmm.*

The analysis that follows considers the responses to disorder in terms of the sequential position in the *repair initiation opportunity space* (Schegloff, Jefferson, & Sacks, 1977). The *repair initiation opportunity space* spans three turns at talk including the space immediately following the trouble source turn which may be extended in order to allow further opportunity for self-repair, i.e., self-correction:

- Trouble source turn—(e.g., disorder) speaker A
- Transition space following trouble source—speaker A
- Next turn—(e.g., collusion, no response, repair initiation) speaker B
- Third turn—speaker A

Self-Repair

Data show Dana to be a highly skilled conversationalist. Further evidence is shown in her ability to carry out self-repairs.

Extract 5: (8.6) LML1-3.272

```
01.    Dana:    #no:# the children: the children I mean the
02.             school's packed with kids .hhh but- n they all
03.             come up n down the stree:t,
```

Dana is talking about the children who walk past her house on their way to and from school. In line 1, she begins with "the children," which is repeated followed by an explicit repair marker *I mean*. Dana then redesigns the turn making the school the subject of the utterance and the sheer number of children forms the description of the school: "packed with kids" (line 2). A further self-repair follows, in line 2, as Dana extends her turn using the conjunction *but*. This is cut off and replaced with *and* which is a more fitted conjunction for the assertion that the children "coming up and down the street" is additional information and not in opposition to the "school being packed with kids."

The example illustrates how finely tuned turn design is at both the topic and syntactic levels. That Dana retains and uses abilities to do self-repair on both these levels evidences how important it is for persons with dementia to make themselves understood.

Self-Repair Following a Delayed Response

By delaying response, second speakers can signal trouble in the previous speaker's turn of talk. The space immediately after the trouble source forms the prime location for an interlocutor to indicate a problem through silence, what Schegloff et al. (1977) describe as the repair initiation opportunity space. After such silence, first speakers can inspect their own, just completed, turns for potential problems and carry out necessary repairs (Pomerantz, 1984). As we have seen, Dana can carry out self-initiated self-repair within her own turn (Extract 5), and in Extract 6, when her interlocutor delays, Dana can attend to this very subtle signal and complete a self-repair.

Extract 6: LML1-11.3003

01.		((30 seconds lapse))
02.	Dana:	so what are you gonna eat
03.		(3.8)
04.	Dana:	what are you gonna eat (.) foryur tea
05.		(0.7)
06.	John:	↓<lasagne>↓
07.		(0.3)
08.	Dana:	Lasagna

Dana's query of her and John's evening meal (line 2) is the fourth time in 40 minutes that she has asked this. John's three times response has no doubt had an effect on the design, timing, and delivery of this fourth response: John delays, extending the transition space to a considerable 3.8 seconds. Dana pursues a response, repeating the question. When no immediate response from John comes in the micropause in line 4, Dana repairs with the clarifying phrase "for yur tea."[4] Dana's repair is successful and prompts a response from John (line 6).

Although we have Dana attending to repair in the transition space of Extract 6, importantly, no repairs occurred in relation to the delusion expressed in Extract 4 despite transition space opportunity. So, it seems that while Dana's conversational competence is such that she can easily recognize subtle practices of cuing topic or syntactic repair; delayed responses are not sufficient to prompt a self-repair on delusion or nonfactual talk.

Thinking Points

- Persons with dementia in this and other research findings are shown to retain the ability to self-repair interactional practices.
- They can sometimes recognize perceptual cues (e.g., significant delays or no response) from their interlocutors that signify trouble within previous turns and then conduct appropriate self-repair (e.g., clarifications, syntax, change in topic focus).
- However, despite the opportunity to do so, the person with dementia above does *not* use self-repair to correct those turns of talk that are delusional or nonfactual.

Question: How might knowing these details facilitate better interactions with persons with dementia?

Other-Initiated Repair

A range of repair initiators are available to interlocutors who perceive an error. They can choose not to initiate repair through delayed turns (i.e., silence), as seen above. Alternatively, repair can be initiated through a

[4]It is the habit of Northern British speakers to refer to the evening meal as "tea."

repeat or partial repeat of the trouble source turn. Extract 7 is a short extract in which John employs a repeat after Dana refers to her late husband in the present.

Extract 7: LML1-11.2450

01.	Dana:	your dah's still in be:d j'know
02.		(0.4)
03.	John:	me dad
04.		(1.1)
05.	Dana:	your dad's dea:d
06.		(0.2)
07.	John:	yea.
08.	Dana:	HA HA ha hahaha

Following Dana's turn in line 1, John repeats the referent of Dana's utterance "me dad." By producing this repeat, the trouble source is located but no specific error is identified. In line 5, Dana demonstrates her knowledge that her husband (John's father) is dead.

One of the typical uses of a repeated turn is as an understanding check (Schegloff et al., 1977, p. 379). John's repeat, therefore, could have been taken as an understanding check, repeated for Dana to confirm the referent. If so, she might have said, *yes, your dad.* Since John offers no explicit contradiction to the disordered talk in Extract 7, no blame is attached to the speaker regarding the trouble source turn. This interactional choice can be optimal in that if the repair initiation fails to prompt the recipient to revise the disordered reality, then the repair initiator can be retracted or sequentially deleted (i.e., essentially ignored or dismissed). John's repeat, as repair initiator, has deflected the need for him to overtly deal with the error. Since Dana does take up the repair initiator by revising her state of reality (line 5), her lapse in competence has been exposed. This is modulated by her laughter in line 8. Such laughter in conversations between non-impaired interlocutors[5] has been characterized as troubles-resistant laughter in which the trouble is played off as a joke or humorous, demonstrating speakers' resilience

[5]This competency has also been noted in stroke victims, see Wilkinson (1995).

to their errors (Jefferson, 1984; Schegloff et al., 1977, p. 378). Dana's response demonstrates her competency to recognize cues of trouble, respond to them, and to laugh off errors as humorous.

In mundane conversations between unimpaired participants, a recipient of a perceived error need not initiate or carry out repair (i.e., correction); as Schegloff et al. (1977, p. 375) note, "even the 'ripest' of repairables [...] are not necessarily followed by repair." When conversing with a person with dementia who may have difficulty keeping track of what has been said in earlier turns, an interlocutor's use of a repair initiator (in the above extracts, a "repeat") keeps the trouble source in focus by re-presenting the utterance. Since no explicit contradiction has been uttered, no blame is attached to the speaker of the trouble source turn at the point when the repair initiator is produced. If it is not recognized as a repair initiator, then it can be retracted without exposing the incongruous reality. Furthermore, by producing the repair initiator, the interlocutor has used the conversational slot (Schegloff et al., 1977) where the co-participant might be expected to align with the disorder. Whatever the outcome of the repair initiation, the co-participant has, thereby, avoided aligning or disaligning with the disordered talk. This practice shows that contradicting a person's "reality" can be carried out in delicate ways that avoid agreeing with everything that the person with dementia says while also restoring the person to a congruous reality by capitalizing on retained competence.

Thinking Points

- Persons with dementia may retain the interactional competence to recognize co-participant repeats (e.g., "me dad," Extract 7) that signal trouble in previous turns of talk.
- When recognized, the person with dementia has the opportunity to repair the trouble and to retain a sense of interactional dignity and personhood.
- If the person with dementia fails to recognize the repeat as an other-initiated repair, no foreseeable negative outcome such as undue stress is expected.

Interlocutor Responses to Disordered Talk: Correction

Correction is understood to be a sub-type of repair and is "commonly understood to be the replacement of an 'error' or 'mistake' with what is 'correct'" (Schegloff et al., 1977, p. 363). In ordinary conversation, Schegloff et al. (1977) observe that the incidence of "correction" is rare, and when it does occur, there are particular practices relating to the design and sequential placing of these cases. For example, corrections in typical talk are invariably modulated. Methods of modulating may include humor or a correction that includes uncertainty markers ("well, I'm not sure, but I think …"). Additionally, one may modulate by accounting, such as giving an explanation for an interlocutor's error (oh, that's okay, it was so long ago, and I can hardly keep those dates straight, either). When unmodulated corrections do occur, according to Schegloff, they are overwhelmingly found to be following a prior attempt at either a modulated correction or an understanding check (e.g., Person A: We eat dinner at four. Person B: At four?) Being atypical, a correction deviates from expected conversation patterns and this unexpectedness could cause distress in the person with dementia.

Extract 8 provides an example in which the unimpaired interlocutors George and his wife, Trudy, have made several attempts to help their mother remember a location that they, apparently, expect that she should remember. As the conversation continues, George seems frustrated and responds to his mother with an unmodulated response, or correction.

Extract 8: LML7-3.15166

01.	George:	it was called Safeway when you used to shop
02.		it's called Morrisons now
03.	Dana:	and where is it
04.	Trudy:	in Horcombe!
05.		((1.0) *eating*))
06.	Trudy:	just past the li'l- all the shops
07.		((3.6) *eating*))
08.	Trudy:	you used to drive me<sometimes when you used
09.		to drive>
10.	George:	@just off Blunt Street where Horcombe working

11.		mens club is,@
12.		((5.6) *eating*))
13.	Dana:	°°(ah dunno:)°°
14.	George:	=>i' dunt matter if you<can't remember
15.		(.)
16.	George:	dunt matter
17.	Trudy:	@it was a long time ago now@(.) since
18.		[you've been dri:ving]
19.	Dana:	[w'l- WHICH roa:d i]s it o:n that would be
20.		more functional=
21.	George:	=@uv just told yu Blunt Street@
22.		(.)
23.	Dana:	Blunt Street in Ho:rcombe

George's interactional choices are a rare instance in these data of an interlocutor drawing attention to the person with dementia's disorder (in this case, faulty memory). George shows his exasperation, in line 21, saying "I've just told you, Blunt Street," after his mother's challenge in lines 19 and 20 "w'l- WHICH roa:d is it on, that would be more functional."

This lack of modulation contrasts with George's earlier attempt to either change the subject or, perhaps, to minimize the interactional tension ("it don't matter if you can't remember" … "don't matter," lines 14, 16). Dana's emphasis on "WHICH" and her not-so-subtle insinuation ("that would be more functional," lines 19–20) that her interlocutors have not been specific enough suggest that Dana, too, is frustrated by the conversation. Note, also, that she does not acknowledge George's suggestion that her memory is to blame; to the contrary, she seems to be countering that suggestion. In any case, it does seem clear that trouble is occurring in the conversation. A potential way to avoid or minimize this trouble is to respond to repeated requests "as if for the first time" and include both modulation and accountings (Jones, 2012, p. 194). After George's emphasis on his mother's lack of memory, Trudy moves this direction from repeated statements of fact that attempt to fill in the missing memory to modulate and account for that lack of memory ("it was a long time ago now since you've been driving," lines 17–18). By line 23 Dana acknowledges receipt that the conversation has been about "Blunt Street, in Horcombe."

In contrast to the above attempts to correct faulty memory, the next example shows an attempt to correct misperception and fear. It is not always prudent or possible for co-participants to simply agree or go along with disordered talk (or perceptions) of persons with dementia within their care. In these data, other-initiated other-corrections *can* occur as modulated repairs that also, from an observer's perspective, demonstrate respect for the concerns or fears of the person with dementia. The following extract presents such a case. The son John quickly initiates a modulating response. This type of other-initiated correction can demonstrate respect for the concerns or fears of the person with dementia. Like many folks, Dana has worries or concerns which need to be addressed in daily conversation. Some concerns involve her personal safety, and many involve her fear regarding large trees and telegraph poles, which she can see from her sitting room. Extracts 9 and 10 show how Dana's co-participants choose interactional strategies that allow them to contradict her perceptions while simultaneously allaying her concerns and fears.

Extract 9: LML5-6.12026

01.	Dana:	an h- ho:w Elsie's gonna get rid of tha' tree
02.		I do not know
03.		(0.3)
04.	John:	((LS)) (0.3) big innit
05.		(.)
06.	Dana:	she's letting it get big[ger an bigger] an ↑big↑ger=
07.	John:	[((*cough*))]
08.	Dana:	an it's gonna fall an kill somebody
09.		(0.6)
10.	John:	h.) a don't think it'll fall over that tree mam
11.		(.)
12.	Dana:	don't you think so?
13.	John:	it's got a nice big trunk to it (h) (0.4)

Dana expresses fears that the large tree she can see in her neighbor's garden will "fall and kill somebody" (line 8). John contradicts this perception with a turn-initial uncertainty marker "I don't think" (line 10).

By selecting this uncertainty marker, John both presents his dissent but also acknowledges that "falling trees" is a real-life possibility, which shows respect to his mother's fear. John's disagreement with his mother's assessment is made stronger in his formulation "that tree" will not fall over. This strong dissent is mitigated with his choice of the turn-final address term *mam*. Modulating his disagreement, his correction of his mother's view, using the familial address term "mam" (or mum), invokes respect and "doing *speaking from the heart*" (Clayman, 2010, original emphasis).

John provides additional support, or an account, for his view in line 13, stating that the reason that tree will not fall and kill someone is because "it's got a nice big trunk to it." He provides evidence that this tree is stable. The way in which John formulated his contradiction, or correction, of Dana's perception on this subject both validates that her fear is real and reassures her that the tree will not fall.

Coupland, Coupland, and Giles, in their review of discourse with elderly patients, note that it is important to acknowledge the real distress that patients express. To deflect or deny they are experiencing problems or fears is to deny those people the "health- and identity-bolstering of supportive discourse" (1991, p. 190). That is, in this instance, if John were to present a version of reality that removed all possibility of the tree falling, this would refute Dana's perception completely, casting her worry as absurd. By formulating the contradicting turn to accept the possibility of trees falling and associated fears, John is giving a credible account of his perception of reality, that this tree will not fall, and supporting his mother's identity as a rational person.

In extract 10, Dana and John are discussing the telegraph pole and cables which can be seen from her window. Dana expresses concerns that the pole could fall. As discussed above, Dana's cognitive impairment seems to inhibit her rationalizing such fears, debilitating her ability to call upon her life experience and knowledge, i.e., a significant proportion of the pole is unseen underground and gives it stability.

Extract 10: LML4-3.10484

01.	Dana:	(°right°) I don't like it there (.) because if
02.		the bloody thing fell it would wreck ↓this↓ joint
03.		(2.7)
04.	Dana:	it would>it would<wreck this house,
05.		(2.2)
06.	John:	w-) it ↑cant↑ fa:ll °mam° (.) >even if- even if<it
07.		was (0.4) broken ↑off↑ at the bottom.
08.		(1.4)
09.	John:	it couldn' fall one way or the>other
10.		be[cause of the<cables]
11.	Dana:	[oh: is it] is it ↑stee:l↑ inside.
12.	John:	↑no↑ because of the cables attached to it'ud
13.		(.) they'd hold it in position ↓more or↓
14.		less [it'd]=
15.	Dana:	[oh:]
16.	John:	=it' tilt ↑over↑ one way but (0.4) it wouldn' go far

Dana expresses her fears about the pole falling onto her house in lines 1–2. When John fails to respond for a considerable 2.7 seconds, Dana repeats her concern "it would, it would wreck this house" (line 4). In line 5, a further pause of 2.2 seconds occurs before John responds. John's turn is formulated as a certainty "it can't fall" (line 6), but this turn is again modulated with the endearment term *mam*. So although John has not weakened this assertion with certainty markers, he gives a detailed account of why he thinks the pole is stable: that the cables would "hold it in position" so that it "wouldn't go far." As in the previous Extract (9), John has formulated his contradiction with a balance between acknowledging the possibility that a pole could get broken and disputing that it would fall onto her house. He seems to have achieved alignment between validating his mother's fears as real and assuaging them.

In the following Extract (11), Dana proposes that she could go to her hairdressing appointment by bus, which is what she did habitually for many years before the progression of dementia prevented this. Some of Dana's regular activities have been able to continue due to the support of her family and, indeed, members of the local community including her hairdresser. Relying on the bus for transportation, however, is not a practice that is safe any longer.

Extract 11: LML1-3.58

01.	John:	'am taking you to the hairdressers
02.		(0.3)
03.	Dana:	>why<
04.		(0.5)
05.	Dana:	I get'n on the bus
06.	John:	y' can't get on the bus mam
07.		(.).
08.	Dana:	why.
09.		(.)
10.	John:	because they don't run up here anymore

Although John has been driving his mother to her regular weekly appointment for some time, Dana is surprised by this and insists she can go by bus (line 5). John immediately corrects this assumption in line 6 appended with the familiar endearment term, *mam*. The ambiguity of the modal verb *can* produces alternative possible meanings for John's turn, relating to its epistemic meaning of permission or deontic meaning of ability (Levinson, 1983); thus, it may be ambiguous whether John is forbidding his mother to get on the bus or stating that she is not able to. He does not, however, offer an account for this until Dana asks *why*. John's response in line 10 provides the sufficient account and resolves the ambiguity of *can*: John's objection is not of Dana's personal ability but, rather, to the ability of any local traveler because the buses "don't run up here anymore."

Extract 11, again, demonstrates circumstances where Dana's interlocutor was compelled to correct her disordered assumptions. On this occasion, Dana's personal safety may be at risk if John allowed her to believe she could take the bus to the hairdressing salon. As seen in Extracts 9, 10, and 11, Dana's emotional well-being was protected as she expressed concerns about her own safety. John's account of why Dana cannot get on the bus is, perhaps, serendipitous since it would not be safe for Dana to travel without assistance. John has exploited the recent changes in local bus routes to truthfully avoid telling Dana that she is no longer competent to travel alone. Dana's interlocutors frequently repair, or correct, misunderstandings based on trying "the least complicated and costly remedy first" (Pomerantz, 1984, p. 156); in doing so, they can correct the conversational disorder without exposing her medical disorder.

Thinking Points

- Corrections can come across as unexpected and cause trouble in conversation.
- Corrections in typical talk are invariably modulated. Try humor; uncertainty markers ("well, I'm not sure, but I think..."); accounting, such as giving an explanation.
- It is possible to acknowledge fears or concerns of the person with dementia, even if they are unwarranted, yet sometimes still successfully offer a correction.

Questions to ponder: Must every error of fact or misunderstanding be corrected? Is contradicting or disagreeing with the person with dementia necessarily corrective? Does a given correction serve a necessary purpose? If so, can it be done without being patronizing or otherwise treating the person as a child, in a way that respects the personhood of the one corrected?

Summary

The data show that co-participants can often respond to disordered talk without detriment to the person with dementia (e.g., evidence of stress) and, sometimes, facilitate competence in interaction. The conversation strategies of alignment, repair initiation, and correction, all of which occur in mundane conversation, can be put to productive use and may allow opportunity for any retained conversational competence on the part of the person with dementia to emerge. This competence can unexpectedly arise even during times of otherwise confused or disordered talk. These strategies demonstrate ways in which conversation can be conducted and facilitated while still respecting a person's perspective, dignity, and personhood.

Aligning through the use of minimal tokens, generalized responses, or collusion can often allow for the progression of talk or can trigger self-correction from the person with dementia. Aligning with disordered talk can go off without trouble, but we also saw John entering into Dana's disordered perspective with the talk of the photograph which left him stranded in that unreality. Still, Dana's momentary recovery of the reality did not appear to have detrimental effects in their interaction. Likewise, when Dana returned to the disordered view that the images in the photograph were actual people, John's attempt to correct her view was not effective. These strategies seem to fit with interactional practices noted in mundane conversations of non-impaired persons: attempt the easiest solution first (Pomerantz, 1984; Svennevig, 2008). In this way, the propensity during typical talk to apply strategies in which no blame for interactional troubles is ascribed to participants also applies to talk with people with dementia.

Similarly, since a preference for self-repair exists in mundane conversation (Schegloff et al., 1977), co-participants should feel confident in using interactional cues to signal *repairables*, or areas of trouble, resulting from cognitive impairment. The data show persons with dementia are able to recognize these interactional cues well into the progression of disease. Strategies of delayed response and of using repeats can expose the trouble in the conversation and trigger a repair without being disrespectful to the personhood of the interlocutor. The advantages of adopting these ordinary approaches to interactional trouble in our interactions with persons with dementia are twofold:

1. The trouble is resolved without undue disruption to the conversation, minimizing the potential for the person with dementia to feel a loss of dignity or personhood (i.e., experience face threating action, see Brown & Levinson, 2006; Goffman, 1967).
2. Conversational partners are treating the person with dementia as fully competent participants (Goffman, 1968).

In everyday interaction, situations arise in which the co-participant, particularly the carer, needs to correct moments of disordered talk or confusion. For example, worries, fears, or potentially harmful occurrences must often be addressed. In such cases in the data, the conversational partners are best served when the co-participant validates the anxiety or intention (e.g., to get on a bus) of the person with dementia and then contradicts the proposition entailed in the turn, often with modulation. Such modulation may occur with the use of endearment terms, with accounting and often with humor, which are, again, the very characteristics that Schegloff et al. (1977) noted in ordinary talk when interlocutors correct others.

Practical Highlights

1. Many of the strategies used by unimpaired co-participants within mundane conversations are recognized by and facilitate competence in persons with dementia: alignment, repair, and correction practices.
2. As in mundane conversation, strategies may have unexpected consequences. Thus, careful monitoring of the conversation for such things as trouble or displays of stress can help the co-participant best facilitate the person with dementia's competence.
3. When trouble arises or strategies fail, it is key for the non-impaired conversation partner to temper urges to defend one's own actions and to refrain from arguing, patronizing, or otherwise treating the person with dementia as a child.
4. It is also important to remember that interaction—even the occasional troubled one—is one way to keep the person with dementia engaged and it provides opportunity for expressions of personhood.

References

Blum, N. S. (1994). Deceptive practices in managing a family member with Alzheimer's disease. *Symbolic Interaction, 17*(1), 21–36.

Brown, P., & Levinson, S. C. (2006). Politeness: Some universals in language usage. In A. Jaworski & N. Coupland (Eds.), *The discourse reader* (2nd ed., pp. 321–335). London, UK: Routledge.

Clayman, S. E. (2010). Address terms in the service of other actions: The case of news interview talk. *Discourse and Communication, 4*(2), 161–183.

Coupland, N., Coupland, J., & Giles, H. (1991). *Language, society and the elderly: discourse, identity and ageing*. Oxford, UK: Blackwell.

Day, A. M., James, I. A., Meyer, T. D., & Lee, D. R. (2011). Do people with dementia find lies and deception in dementia care acceptable? *Aging and Mental Health, 15*(7), 822–829.

Goffman, E. (1967 [1955]). On face-work. In E. Goffman (Ed.), *Interaction ritual: Essays on face-to-face behavior* (pp. 33–40). New York, NY: Pantheon Books.

Goffman, E. (1968 [1963]). *Stigma: Notes on the management of spoiled identity*. Harmondsworth, UK: Penguin.

Guendouzi, J., & Müller, N. (2006). *Approaches to discourse in dementia*. Mahwah, NJ: Lawrence Erlbaum.

Hamilton, H. E. (1994). *Conversations with an Alzheimer's patient: An interactional sociolinguistic study*. Cambridge, UK: Cambridge University Press.

Jefferson, G. (1984). Laughter organization in talk about troubles. In J. M. Atkinson & J. Heritage (Eds.), *Structures of social action: Studies in conversation analysis* (pp. 346–369). Cambridge, UK: Cambridge University Press.

Jones, D. (2012). *Family conversations with an Alzheimer's sufferer: A conversation analytic study*. Unpublished Ph.D. thesis, University of York, UK.

Levinson, S. C. (1983). *Pragmatics*. Cambridge, UK: Cambridge University Press.

Lindholm, C. (2015). Parallel realities: The interactional management of confabulation in dementia care encounters. *Research on Language and Social Interaction, 48*(2), 176–199.

Lindley, L. M. (2016). *Competence in everyday interaction: A conversation analytic approach to repetition, confusion and getting things done when living with dementia*. Ph.D. thesis, University of Leeds, UK. http://etheses.whiterose.ac.uk/id/eprint/14314.

Mikesell, L. (2009). Conversational practices of a frontotemporal dementia patient and his interlocutors. *Research on Language and Social Interaction, 42*(2), 135–162.

Mok, Z., & Müller, N. (2014). Staging casual conversations for people with dementia. *Dementia, 13*(6), 834–853.

Müller, N., & Guendouzi, J. A. (2005). Order and disorder in conversation: Encounters with dementia of the Alzheimer's type. *Clinical Linguistics & Phonetics, 19*(5), 393–404.

Perkins, L., Whitworth, A., & Lesser, R. (1998). Conversing in dementia: A conversation analytic approach. *Journal of Neurolinguistics, 11*(1–2), 33–53.

Pomerantz, A. (1984). Pursuing a response. In J. M. Atkinson & J. Heritage (Eds.), *Structures of social action: Studies in conversation analysis* (pp. 152–163). Cambridge, UK: Cambridge University Press.

Potter, J. (1996). *Representing reality: Discourse, rhetoric and social construction.* London, UK: Sage.

Quince, C. (2011). *Support, stay, save: Care and support of people with dementia in their own homes.* London, UK: Alzheimer's Society.

Sabat, S. R., & Lee, J. M. (2011). Relatedness among people diagnosed with dementia: Social cognition and the possibility of friendship. *Dementia, 11*(3), 315–327.

Schegloff, E. A., Jefferson, G., & Sacks, H. (1977). The preference for self-correction in the organization of repair in conversation. *Language, 53*(2), 361–382.

Svennevig, J. (2008). Trying the easiest solution first in other-initiation of repair. *Journal of Pragmatics, 40,* 333–348.

Tuckett, A. G. (2012). The experience of lying in dementia care: A qualitative study. *Nursing Ethics, 19*(1), 7–20.

Wardaugh, R., & Fuller, J. M. (2015). *An introduction to sociolinguistics* (2nd ed.). Chichester, UK: Wiley-Blackwell.

Wilkinson, R. (1995). Doing 'being ordinary': Aphasia as a problem of interaction. In *Department of Human Communication Science work in progress* (Vol. 5, pp. 131–150). London, UK: Department of Human Communication Science, University College London.

Recommended Readings

Antaki, C. (2011). Six kinds of applied conversation analysis. In C. Antaki (Ed.), *Applied conversation analysis: Intervention and change in institutional talk* (pp. 1–14). Basingstoke, UK: Palgrave Macmillan.

Magnusson, S. (2014). *Where memories go: Why dementia changes everything.* London, UK: Two Roads.

Phillipson, L., & Hammond, A. (2018). More than talking: A scoping review of innovative approaches to qualitative research involving people with dementia. *International Journal of Qualitative Methods, 17,* 1–13.

Schegloff, E. A., Jefferson, G., & Sacks, H. (1977). The preference for self-correction in the organization of repair in conversation. *Language, 53*(2), 361–382.

8

Meaningfulness at the Intersection of Knowledge and Environmental Objects: Investigating Interactions in Art Galleries and Residences Involving Persons with Dementia and Their Carers

Adrienne R. Isaac and Heidi E. Hamilton

Learning Objectives

By the end of this chapter, you will be able to:

- Better understand how objects in the immediate physical environment can be used to foster interactional meaningfulness with individuals with dementia;

The authors wish to thank Trini Stickle and an anonymous reviewer for their insightful comments on a previous version of the manuscript.

A. R. Isaac (✉) · H. E. Hamilton
Department of Linguistics, Georgetown University, Washington, DC, USA
e-mail: ari6@georgetown.edu

H. E. Hamilton
e-mail: hamilthe@georgetown.edu

T. Stickle (ed.), *Learning from the Talk of Persons with Dementia*,
The Language of Mental Health, https://doi.org/10.1007/978-3-030-43977-4_8

- View meaningful discursive practices in which agency and authority are afforded to individuals with dementia, particularly by allowing them to initiate questions related to their own interests and by asking them questions about their own lives;
- Practice meaningful discourse strategies centered on immediately present objects in public spaces (e.g., care facility hallways and dining rooms) and private spaces (e.g., private rooms) that you might use as a conversational partner with an individual with dementia;
- Practice being a discourse analyst by evaluating actual conversations with individuals with dementia and their visitors by identifying discourse strategies that advance or inhibit conversations and proposing alternative strategies where applicable.

Introduction

Micro-analytic studies over the past three decades documenting the real-time details of human interactions have illuminated ways in which objects in the environment may play a mutually elaborative role in the shaping of unfolding interaction. In particular, such artifacts have been shown to facilitate the display and demonstration of knowledge (Aaltonen, Arminen, & Raudaskoski, 2014; Goodwin, 1994, 2013; Nevile, Haddington, Heinemann, & Rauniomaa, 2014).

In this chapter, we consider how discursive practices centered on objects have the potential to enhance the well-being of persons with dementia. In Section 1, we examine the language used within an art gallery program involving guides who are specially trained to work with visitors with dementia. Specifically, we investigate knowledge asymmetries (Heritage, 2012) within question-answer sequences, focusing on two types of interactions in which paintings are used to promote interactional meaningfulness: (1) those in which visitors pose questions to guides that relate to the visitors' *own* interests; and (2) those in which guides pose questions to visitors regarding topics that relate to the visitors' personal lives. We argue that the former type of interaction affords the visitors personal agency, while the latter type of interaction allows them to display their authoritative knowledge. In Section 2, then, we guide the reader through a series of pedagogical exercises that center on local objects found in assisted living facilities; in these exercises, the reader has the opportunity to assume the roles of both a potential conversational partner and a discourse analyst, and experiences first-hand how meaningful conversations might be sparked by the environment in both public and private spaces of these care homes. These activities share the common goal of the discourse practices that we explore in the first part of the chapter; i.e., to enhance the well-being of persons with dementia.

Background

A burgeoning area of research within the field of human interaction has centered on processes of meaning-making that result from the reflexive relationship between unfolding interaction and the material surround (e.g., Goodwin, 1994, 2000, 2013, 2017; Nevile et al., 2014; Streeck, Goodwin, & LeBaron, 2011). Interactionally local objects, in particular, have been found to serve as rich sites toward which participants' mutual attention can be directed, and can serve as focal points for both talk and indexical gestures (Streeck et al., 2011). Nevile et al. (2014) argue that objects "are constitutive of and constituted through interactions" (p. 4), differentiating objects as *situated resources* (how objects are used by participants in interaction) from objects as *practical accomplishments* (how objects are oriented to and shaped by participants through interaction). Objects in the environment can center meaningful engagement in that they can be used "to augment communication, and to afford participation and action" (Nevile et al., 2014, p. 15); in particular, they may interact with an individual's "extroverted" consciousness (Chafe, 1994, p. 38) as it engages with the immediate physical environment by *perceiving, acting*, and *evaluating*, or with an individual's "introverted" consciousness as it engages in a more displaced way by *remembering* and *imagining*. Finally, physical objects represent the "present extra-verbal, situational locale" (Bergmann, 1990, p. 207) or the "local sensitivity" of a conversational sequence.

As Nevile et al. (2014) note, objects can be invoked within interaction to claim or demonstrate knowledge. A "perspicuous" (Garfinkel & Wieder, 1992, p. 184) physical setting at the intersection of concrete environmental artifacts and the display of knowledge is the art gallery. In such settings, visitors have been observed "...constitute[ing] the sense and significance of the images, objects and artefacts" (vom Lehn, Heath, & Hindmarsh, 2005, p. 231) through their action and interaction. Important related efforts by analysts to understand the role of knowledge within such settings—in particular "... the various ways in which participants in interaction design their contributions, and understand the contributions of others, in relation to a distribution of knowledge that is assumed to preexist" (Sidnell, 2015, p. 1)—fall within what is referred to as the epistemics of social interaction (see also Heritage, 2012; Stivers, Mondada, & Steensig, 2011). This research area has focused its efforts on how interlocutors orient to knowledge differences in the way they order utterances within a sequence, design their utterances and engage in action formation (Heritage, 2012; Heritage & Raymond, 2005). With respect to the knowledge asymmetries that play out in such patterns of interaction, the participant with relatively greater epistemic access to a particular knowledge domain is said to have greater *epistemic status* (Heritage, 2012).

Within institutional settings, expectations regarding the distinct roles of representatives and clients correspond with role-structured asymmetries related to knowledge rights and participation across the two participant groups. Indeed, it has long been understood (e.g., Agar, 1985; Drew & Heritage, 1992) that representative-client social interaction is relatively constrained, making certain contributions more allowable than others with respect to the particular work at hand. Drew and Heritage (1992, p. 39) refer to "specialized institutional turn-taking systems" that influence such conversational features as turn design and sequence organization.

From a discourse analytic perspective, such knowledge asymmetries can be viewed through the lens of an institution's discourse ecology which "...sets limits around what either the institutional representative or the client can do during institutional discourse" (Agar, 1985, p. 158). As Agar argues, it is within such ecologies that institutional representatives control information flow primarily through their use of question-answer sequences. More specifically, the institutional representative "often has the conversational right to ask questions, to initiate (and change) topics, to choose who speaks and when … and more generally to set the interactive agenda" (Freed, 2015).

Question-answer sequences, in particular, have garnered the attention of researchers in the way they display asymmetries in the distribution of, and rights to, knowledge between institutional and lay participants. In these sequences, institutional representatives typically maintain greater knowledge regarding the topics of talk and exercise greater discursive control over the trajectory of the interaction than do the lay participants (Drew & Heritage, 1992; Freed, 2015; Freed & Ehrlich, 2010; Heritage & Clayman, 2010). In this way, institutional representatives enact their "institution-relevant identities" (Heritage, 2004, p. 106) as they carry out their agenda, either by asking what Searle (1969) has called *known-answer* questions or requesting that lay participants provide information relevant to the pursuit of an institutional goal.

For the purposes of the present chapter, the art gallery setting in which physically present objects in the form of paintings prompt and support visitor displays of knowledge is particularly well-suited for individuals who are managing intermediate-term (Kesner & Hunsaker, 2010) episodic memory and word-finding difficulties that are typically associated with early stages of dementia, especially of the Alzheimer's type (Hamilton, 2019; Hodges, 2000; Shelley-Tremblay, 2011). Indeed, the immediate physical environment has been found to play a large role in the structuring of discourse among persons with dementia; e.g., Hamilton (2008) found that the majority of talk involving an individual with Alzheimer's disease centered on physical objects or people in the immediate environment rather than involving memories or abstract thoughts. Furthermore, when memories were recounted in the form of short narratives or narrative traces, these seemed to be sparked by objects in the immediate physical environment. These findings may be explained by the phenomenon of *context-boundedness* (Appell, Kertesz, & Fisman, 1982; Obler, 1981), characterized by Hamilton (2008, pp. 63–64) as an "…individual's reduced ability to free him- or herself cognitively from the immediate temporal and spatial context" (see also Hamilton, 2019, pp. 159–172 for more information).

Data

The data analyzed in this chapter come from a research study involving guided tours at a major art gallery in Australia with participants who had been diagnosed with dementia. The goal of the initial study in which these recordings were made was to explore the degree to which persons with dementia were able to engage with artwork in an art gallery setting, as well as the extent to which the program affected their well-being given the appropriate facilitation to do so. More specifically, the original study "was based on work by Artists for Alzheimer's (ARTZ) in the USA (Zeisel, 2009), which aims to promote quality of life for people with dementia by providing an intellectually stimulating environment in which they are actively engaged with other people and with artworks" (MacPherson, Bird, Anderson, Davis, & Blair, 2009, p. 745). The specially trained guides were asked to shift their usual focus from teaching about the paintings to "encourage[ing] the participants to express what they see and feel about the art" (Zeisel, 2009, p. 98). Given this institutional support for extended discussion among visitors, then, the gallery tours examined in this chapter differ significantly from usual tours in which visitors congregate silently around a painting while a gallery guide provides details about the artwork.

This larger study consisted of twelve video-recorded sessions involving sixteen individuals, half of whom were in the early stages of dementia, and half of whom were in later stages of the disease. Group determinations were made based on relative stage of the disease (see also Hamilton, 2011; MacPherson et al., 2009 for a description of these data). The guided tours lasted approximately an hour each, as four or five paintings were viewed in succession. Discussion sessions were facilitated by the physical layout of the interactional space. In all sessions, visitors sat on a bench or in wheelchairs in front of the artwork. The lead guide typically stood next to the painting while one to two additional guides sat in chairs next to the visitors on either side of the bench. The guides who sat with the visitors attempted to assume the visitors' visual perspective and often attended to the visitors' overlapping talk, both to which the lead guide may not have had access.

The extracts in this chapter were taken from three hour-long tours involving visitors in the early stage of dementia, as these visitors exhibited a greater degree of interactional engagement (asking more questions and attending more fully to the guides' questions) than did the visitors in later stages of the disease. Segments of video-recorded interactions in which questions were posed by either a guide or a visitor were identified; we then noted which participant (visitor or guide) could be assumed to have greater authority over the knowledge domain as pertaining to the information requested.

Methods

For the purposes of our investigation, we followed Freed and Ehrlich (2010) who note that a question cannot be defined by any single linguistic criterion (see also Bolinger, 1957). Considering both functional and sequential factors, Freed and Ehrlich (2010, p. 6) define questions as those that "solicit (and/or are treated by the recipient as soliciting) information, confirmation or action (Hultgren & Cameron, 2010)" and "are delivered in such a way as to create a slot for the recipient to produce a responsive turn" (Ford, 2010). Applying this definition to our analysis, we included all utterances with interrogative syntax (yes/no, wh-, tag, and alternate questions) as well as utterances containing verbs of cognition with declarative syntax (e.g., "I wonder what she's thinking about").[1]

The resulting corpus of questions we examined invoked one of two knowledge domains: (1) knowledge related to the paintings in the art gallery; and (2) knowledge deriving from personal experiences of the visitors. Relative distinctions in knowledge status and authority between the interlocutors were determined by the particular knowledge domain

[1]The following counted as one question token: restarts, repeats, or reformulations of an initial question; and multiple questions within a turn that topically cohered. Given our focus on the usefulness of a work of art to center interaction between guides and visitors, we excluded the following question tokens: those used to manage the discussion; other-initiated repairs; questions that did not relate to the task at hand (e.g., "Haven't you watched the show on TV?"); and questions initiated by visitors that were directed to other visitors.

invoked by the question: questions asked by guides and visitors that referenced aspects of the painting (e.g., biographical information about the artist, historical period in which a painting was created, information on a particular painting technique) were deemed to reside within the knowledge domain of the guide, while questions referencing personal experiences of the visitors were deemed to reside within the domain of the visitor.

Section 1: Interactional Agency and Authoritative Knowledge Among Participants in Art Gallery Tours

The resulting intersections of questioner-type (initiated by guide or visitor) and epistemic authority relative to a particular knowledge domain can be found in Table 8.1 below. Cell (a) represents questions initiated by art gallery guides pertaining to knowledge within their own

Table 8.1 Intersections of questioner-type and epistemic authority relative to a particular knowledge domain

	Art gallery guides maintain epistemic authority relative to knowledge domain in question n=156 **81% of total questions**	**Art gallery visitors maintain epistemic authority** relative to knowledge domain in question n=37 **19% of total questions**
Questions initiated by **art gallery guides** n=129 **67% of total questions**	(a) Guide: *Do you think it says something about cultural disharmony?* n=93	(c) Guide: *What- what was that used for?* n=36
Questions initiated by **art gallery visitors** n=64 **33% of total questions**	(b) Visitor: *I can't make out what those things are. Are they birds or?* n=63	(d) Visitor: *Can you tell me why I recognize that painting?* n=1

Source Authors

epistemic domain (*known-answer* questions); cell (b) represents questions initiated by art gallery visitors regarding knowledge within the guides' epistemic domain; cell (c) represents questions initiated by art gallery guides pertaining to knowledge within the visitors' epistemic domain; and cell (d) represents questions initiated by art gallery visitors within their own epistemic domain.

Quantitative analyses reveal that art gallery guides asked 129 of the 193 (67%) questions posed during these three tours, while visitors asked 64 of the 193 questions (33%). Of these 193 questions, 156 (81%) queried something (that could be assumed to be) within a guide's epistemic domain; 37 of these 193 questions (19%) queried an aspect of a visitor's epistemic domain. With regard to the specific intersections of questioner-type and epistemic authority, we note that 93 instances represent cell (a); 63 instances represent cell (b); 36 instances represent cell (c); and 1 instance represents cell (d) (see Table 8.1).

In this chapter, we focus on the intersection of knowledge asymmetry and questioner-type that are found in cells (b) and (c) because they represent interactionally meaningful instances wherein the visitors display interactional agency and epistemic authority, respectively.

Intersection (b): Questions Initiated by Art Gallery Visitors Regarding Knowledge in Which Guides Maintain Greater Knowledge Authority

This section examines a single representative question-answer sequence (of 63 instances) in which a visitor asks the guide a question regarding knowledge that can be assumed to be within the guide's knowledge domain. We argue that this instance reveals the art gallery visitor's interactional agency as she assumes control over the shape of the ensuing talk with the issuing of the question. We note that such an interactional pattern represents what Ainsworth-Vaughn (1998) refers to as a *power-claiming discourse strategy*, as it works against the normative pattern of control in institutional discourse described earlier (Drew & Heritage, 1992; Freed, 2015; Freed & Ehrlich, 2010; Heritage & Clayman, 2010).

In the following exchange, participants are about to discuss Napier Waller's *Christian Waller with Baldur, Undine, and Siren at Fairy Hills*,[2] a large painting that depicts a 1930s-era young woman sitting outside on the grass surrounded by three dogs. Visitor Rhonda poses a question within her response to the guide's initial question regarding the presumed location and activity represented in the painting. In her response to the guide's question, Rhonda makes reference to a specific aspect of the painting, seeking to confirm the identity of an object that she perceives to be a "letter" in the hand of the young woman. Rhonda's question shapes the ensuing talk in this sequence as the guide provides a subsequent response instead of pursuing her initial, more generalized topical trajectory.

Extract 1a[3]

	01.	Guide:	I wonder what you think (.) about (.) where they are. What-
	02.		what is happening?
→	03.	Rhonda:	Don't know I- I- (kind of) want to know what- what is in
→	04.		her hand near the dog. Is it a letter or?
	05.	Guide:	Here?
	06.	Rhonda:	Yes.
	07.	Guide:	Yes I think- I think it's a letter,
	08.		Some people think it's a book but I think it's a letter.
	09.		I think you're- you're spot on Rhonda it's- it's act- actually
	10.		((*Janet nods head*))
	11.	Rhonda:	A [letter°
	12.	Guide:	[From my reading about this it's- it's a letter.
	13.	Rhonda:	It's a letter? (Okay)°

Our analysis of this extract centers on the conditional relevance (Schegloff, 2007) between the guide's question and the visitor's response. The guide initiates the sequence by prompting the visitors to interpret "where they are" (line 1) with the question "what is happening" (lines 1 and 2) in the painting. Notably, Rhonda's response to the guide answers neither of these questions explicitly as she first expresses that she doesn't know in line 3 ("Don't

[2]https://artsearch.nga.gov.au/Detail-LRG.cfm?IRN=49895.

[3]See Appendix for transcription conventions.

know"). Such a response, particularly with the absence of the first-person subject "I," can be seen as a dismissal of the guide's question. Her subsequent "I- I- (kind of) want to know..." is not only a question that she poses of her own volition to confirm the identity of an object that she perceives to be a letter, but one that she expresses with intention as she makes her wants explicit. The content of the guide's and Rhonda's questions differs in terms of abstraction with regard to the interpretation of the painting: while the guide's question asks the visitors to generalize from particularities in the painting, Rhonda's question pertains to one particular object that can be identified visually within the painting.

The reader will note that the guide's initial questions did not select specific aspects of the objects of joint attention in the way that Rhonda's question did. This difference in abstraction between the guide's question and that of Rhonda's is representative of Chafe's (1994) dimensions of a speaker's types of consciousness: Rhonda's "extroverted" consciousness *perceives* an object in the environment, while the guide's question prompts the visitors to engage their "introverted" consciousness by imagining "where they are" and "what is happening" in the painting. Further, Rhonda's question codes the object "in her hand near the dog" (lines 3–4) as the object of knowledge (Goodwin, 1994) and highlights it by offering the candidate response "is it a letter or?" (line 4). Rhonda's coding of specific phenomena in the painting shapes the ensuing discourse by firmly anchoring it to the surrounding environment in a way that the guide's question did not, as it negotiates the identity of specific phenomena in the painting.

Moving away from the content of Rhonda's question, it is noteworthy that Rhonda's question influences the ensuing talk as the guide answers Rhonda's question rather than pursuing her own agenda, demonstrating the lay participant's interactional control of the discourse described earlier (Agar, 1985; Drew & Heritage, 1992; Freed, 2015; Freed & Ehrlich, 2010; Heritage & Clayman, 2010). This evidences the flexibility present in these guided visits for those with dementia in which visitors are afforded opportunities to engage in, and display, agency within the course of their talk.

Intersection (c): Questions Initiated by Art Gallery Guides Involving the Visitors' Knowledge Domain

In Extract 1a we noted that the sequence was initiated by the art gallery guide regarding her own institutional knowledge, despite the fact that the visitor's response countered the progressivity of the sequence and the normative institutional discourse ecology. In this section, we illustrate another exchange initiated by an art gallery guide; in this instance (one of 36 instances), however, the guide's question topicalizes knowledge that is assumed to reside within the visitors' knowledge domain, rather than her own.

While the art gallery guides bring to the interactions specialized knowledge of paintings and artists, the visitors, who are elderly, often have first-hand knowledge of life during the time period depicted in some paintings. As such, in this extract the visitors and guides assume a reversal in the roles that were apparent in the previous extract, one that allows for visitors' displays of knowledge authority in an interactional setting that typically disfavors such forms of participation.

In the following segment, participants are discussing artist Grace Cossington Smith's *Interior in Yellow*[4] a painting that depicts a bedroom with a window typical of an older time period. The guide asks about the utility of the window, after which visitors Darla and Rhonda respond to the guide. An analysis of the guide's subsequent utterances retrospectively reveals her intention to *receive*, rather than to *deliver*, information (Heritage, 2012).

Extract 1b

01.	Guide[1]:	I'm just thinking about the room
02.	Rhonda:	The window [(over the door)
03.	Guide[1]:	[Yeah
04.	Darla:	[Yes that window oh that- that's (taking) my eye ()
05.	Rhonda:	Yeah
06.	Darla:	It's an old- uh- [an old roo::m
07.	Rhonda:	[It's an old ( )

[4] https://nga.gov.au/Exhibition/cossingtonsmith/Detail.cfm?IRN=45746.

	08.	Guide^{1}:	Yes
	09.	Darla:	Because (you) don't do that
	10.	Rhonda:	No (we) don't
→	11.	Guide^{2}:	What- what was that used for?
	12.		What was that [used for?
	13.	Rhonda:	[To fix the light into the room? I presu:::me.
	14.	Guide^{2}:	Did- did it open? Do they?
	15.	Rhonda:	Yes
	16.	Darla:	They were [( ) you could pull em on a cord couldn't you ((*looks to Rhonda*))
	17.		if I remember (at the top of them) this uh- the
	18.		light and- and the air too
	19.	Rhonda:	[Yes yes that's right yeah yes yeah
	20.		Yes yes
→	21.	Guide^{2}:	Oh so you like to- to ventilate the house?
	22.	Rhonda:	((*nods head*))
	23.	Darla:	Um (.) yes

Similar to Extract 1a, the guide opens the sequence with an open-ended prompt for discussion through her invocation of the main entity depicted in the painting—the bedroom—as seen in line 1 ("I'm just thinking about the room"). Later in the sequence, however, Guide^{2} poses a question that refers specifically to the window in the room ("What- what was that used for?") as seen in line 11. Importantly, this topic has been initially introduced by Rhonda in line 2 ("The window (over the door)") and immediately embraced topically by fellow visitor Darla in line 4 ("Yes that window oh that- that's (taking) my eye ( )"). Darla's "Because (you) don't do that" (line 9), in which she makes an assertion directed to a collectivity with the generic "you" pronoun, displays knowledge access and rights to the knowledge domain at hand. Rhonda's subsequent assertion in line 10 involving the first-person plural pronoun "we" in "No (we) don't" then serves to differentiate between the two types of members present, knowing and unknowing, regarding the utility of the window depicted in the painting.

As noted above, in line 11, Guide^{2} initiates the topically related question "What- what was that used for?" which she repeats in line 12 ("What was that used for?"). In line 13, Rhonda provides the response ("To fix the light into the room? I presu:::me") to which Guide^{2} asks a follow-up question, as seen in line 14 ("Did- did it open? Do they?"). In response to this inquiry, Darla explains that one could open the window with the cords: "They were ( ) you could pull em on a cord couldn't you if I remember (at the top of them) this uh- the light and- and the air too" (lines 16–18). In saying this, Darla directs her gaze toward Rhonda, who has also earlier (lines 10 and 15) demonstrated knowledge authority in this knowledge domain, while invoking the tag question "couldn't you" which represents an epistemic downgrade (Heritage, 2012) relative to Rhonda. Rhonda validates Darla's response with her agreement and evaluative tokens in line 19 ("Yes yes that's right yeah yes yeah") and in line 20 ("Yes yes"). Rhonda's validation of Darla's talk retrospectively reinforces her position as one who maintains authoritative knowledge that was initially revealed through Darla's gaze and tag question directed to Rhonda as she sought confirmation of the accuracy of her response.

We then see that the guide's third-position utterance displays a *change-of-state token* as in the "oh"-prefaced follow-up question "Oh so you like to- to ventilate the house?" (line 21). Heritage (1984) notes that such tokens are often found in informing and serve to signal the receipt of new information. Guide[2]'s "oh"-prefaced utterance then additionally serves to reinforce the visitors' authoritative knowledge as well as the guide's ostensive purpose of her questions in lines 11, 12, and 14 as those of *requesting*, rather than *delivering*, information.

It is the guide, then, not the visitor, who undergoes a transformation in knowledge in this instance. Such a process reflects Goodwin's (2013, p. 19) description of how "[d]istributions of knowledge… change in ways that are consequential as action unfolds." In other words, the direction of information flow in this segment is the opposite of what we observed in extract 1a. This guide's inquiry "What was that used for?" is not one that would typically be asked by an institutional representative on behalf of the institution to further its goals; instead it represents the special discourse ecology created specifically for this population of visitors, one in which the visitors with dementia may be allowed to assume agency as they are co-constructed as the ones with authoritative knowledge.

Summary of Section 1

The interactions we examined in this first section highlighted some ways in which the immediate physical environment with its visually accessible objects was used to facilitate the display of agency and knowledge in an art gallery. With specific focus on two interactions characterized by question-answer sequences, we demonstrated how specially trained art gallery guides enacted institutional flexibility by providing visitors with dementia opportunities to exert control over the discourse, change the trajectory of talk initiated by the guides, and ask questions based on their own interests. We also illuminated how these same visitors were interactionally situated as displaying authoritative knowledge when the guides asked them questions about information they assumed the visitors would know. The action motivating the questions—one of requesting, rather than delivering, information—was revealed through the guide's response to the visitors' answers when she indexed the receipt of new information (Heritage, 1984) rather than assessing its accuracy, as would be characteristic of responses to *known-answer* questions.

Our findings suggest how art galleries—and perhaps other kinds of museums—may be used to promote personal agency and feelings of well-being for persons with dementia managing symptoms related to memory and language. Conversations that encourage the initiation of questions and the display of personal knowledge may center on environmental objects about which the persons with dementia are curious and/or over which they may maintain authoritative knowledge. These material environments and conversational contexts may, then, creatively and compassionately lead to increased levels of well-being for persons with dementia as social interaction and individual expression are supported.

Crucially, this potential for interactional meaningfulness need not be limited to the rarified space of the art gallery. Objects in public spaces of residential facilities for persons with dementia—including paintings in hallways and dining rooms or displays of artifacts in residential library collections—may promote opportunities for meaningful discussions that rival those that take place in art galleries. Even more meaningful interactions may be sparked by physical objects found within personal living spaces of persons with dementia—including family photographs, pieces of jewelry, travel souvenirs, and collectibles—that may evoke memories of historical and personal relevance for these individuals. It is to these interactions that we now turn.

Section 2: From the Art Gallery to the Home: The Reader's Turn to Apply and Analyze

In the second section of this chapter, the reader has opportunities to explore these insights through pedagogical activities, first by stepping into the role of a potential conversational partner to consider how conversations might be facilitated by objects in the environment in both public spaces (e.g., hallways and dining rooms) (Activity 1a) and private spaces (e.g., photographs and collectibles) (Activity 1b), and, secondly, by taking on the role of a discourse analyst, evaluating conversations that were recorded inside two residents' apartments (Activity 2a) and comparing them to the art gallery interactions above (Activity 2b).

Pedagogical Exercises: Application and Analysis in Home Settings Using Local Objects

Activity 1a: You're the conversational partner

Using objects in *public spaces* to spark conversation

Let's think about how to translate the findings from the empirical study in the art gallery characterized above to a residential setting. First let's focus on **public spaces**:

- The next time you visit an assisted living facility, dementia care unit, or nursing home, take a notebook along with you. As you move within the public spaces, stroll along the hallways, sit in the dining area and group activity spaces, observe very carefully. What paintings, posters, photographs, symbols, or other objects are on the walls? What objects are on tables or shelves? How might you use these objects to spark a meaningful conversation involving personal agency or knowledge with a small group of residents?

- As you envision this conversation, consider what comments you might use to engage the residents. What questions might you pose? (*What's going on here? What do you see that makes you say that? What more can you find?* [Housen, 1999; Ritchhart, 2007]). Notice if anchoring your talk to specific aspects of the objects facilitates discussion, as we saw in the first part of the chapter. Take time to show genuine interest in residents' comments by asking follow-up questions or adding details from your own perspective. Include occasional pauses to invite residents to say what's on their minds, especially in relation to topics about which they might know a great deal.

Activity 1b: You're the conversational partner

Using objects in *private spaces* to spark conversation

Now let's focus on **private spaces:**

- The next time you are invited into a resident's private space, take time to look around you and compare what you notice with what you observed in the more public parts of the assisted living facility, dementia care unit, or nursing home (in response to the prompt above). Look for objects that are likely to be personally meaningful to the resident. What objects from years ago do you see (books, jewelry, furniture, dishes, vases, toys)? Can you find any items that seem to be handmade (quilts, pillows, paintings)? Do you see any collections (coins, stamps, dolls)? What about photographs that appear to be of family members, friends, pets, homesteads?
- Consider how talking about these personally important objects may differ from conversations that are centered on other publicly shared objects as in Activity 1a, or on art gallery paintings, as examined in the first part of the chapter. What special joy may be sparked? What kinds of displays of knowledge emerge? Alternatively, what face threats might surface in conversations about one of these objects: what if the resident doesn't seem to remember what she thinks she should be able to remember? Resist the temptation to pepper the resident with question after question or comment after comment. Allow her the time to initiate her own contribution; after all, she knows much more about these objects than you do!

Activity 2a: You're the analyst

Evaluating actual conversations between persons with dementia and their visitors

Finally let's examine **language used in conversations** from three extracts that were recorded involving persons with dementia in an assisted living facility and their visitors.[5]

In the extract below, a visitor has come to see Mr. Wayne, a resident with dementia in an assisted living facility in the southeastern United States. The visitor has brought along a nature photo calendar and has just pointed out the photographs that accompany the months of January and February (lines 1–3). As the visitor refers to the month of March, Mr. Wayne begins to speak (lines 5 and 7), linking the bridges depicted in the photograph ("like this") to his memories of aspects of nearby geography ("the lowlands of the Carolinas down there"). Rather than expanding on Mr. Wayne's comment, the visitor evaluates it quickly in line 8 ("That's right.") and moves on to the next month's photograph in line 10 ("And uh this was- these were sunflowers.").

Extract 2a: Photo calendar

01.	Visitor:	Uh this was uh our picture of uh January.
02.		Uh do you remember this one?
03.		This was the February picture.
04.		This was the February picture.
05.	Mr. Wayne:	All these kind of bridges like this cross=
06.	Visitor:	=Yeah
07.	Mr. Wayne:	the lowlands of the Carolinas down there.
08.	Visitor:	That's right.
09.	Mr. Wayne:	Exactly. Yeah.
10.	Visitor:	And uh this was- these were sunflowers.
11.	Mr. Wayne:	Sunflowers.
12.	Visitor:	Right. Right. Yes.

[5]We are grateful to Boyd Davis and Charlene Pope for compiling *The Carolinas Conversation Collection* and generously sharing these interactions with us and many other researchers (see Pope & Davis, 2011).

13.	Mr. Wayne:	We raised them.
14.		Mother did.
15.	Visitor:	I see.
16.		We have the pond.
17.		And- there are these-
18.		I like this picture!
19.		This is a- beautiful meadow.
20.	Mr. Wayne:	Mm hmm.
21.	Visitor:	See the the uh clouds in the sky
22.		You see the trees in the back uh in the background
23.		And here in the front uh this is a beautiful meadow.
24.	Mr. Wayne:	Very nice.

Examine the conversational interaction in Extract 2a, lines 13–20, between Mr. Wayne and the visitor. Do the visitor's contributions in lines 15–19 advance or inhibit the contribution Mr. Wayne made in lines 13–14? Consider what else the visitor might have said in line 15 to lead to a richer, more personally meaningful interaction. Now look back to lines 1–7. What contribution might the visitor have made in line 8 to change the trajectory of the conversation? As you think about these options, you may wish to refer back to extracts 1a and 1b of the art gallery interactions in the first part of the chapter; notice particularly the art gallery guides' contributions in lines 7–10 and 12 in Extract 1a as they positively evaluate the visitor's response relative to their institutional knowledge of what others believe, as well as lines 14 and 21 in Extract 1b, as they position the visitors as the ones with authoritative knowledge regarding a particular subject.

In the extract below, a visitor has come to see Ms. Todd, a woman with dementia who lives in the same assisted living facility as Mr. Wayne from Extract 2a above. In contrast to the interaction represented in Extract 2a, this visitor has not brought a physical object with her; instead, she uses objects (a collection of bells) that are already in Ms. Todd's residence to spark a new topic of conversation.

Note in Extract 2b below how the topic of the bell collection emerges from the previous topic of Ms. Todd's marriage. Then examine subsequent turns-at-talk by both conversationalists to advance this new topic.

Extract 2b: Bell collection (part 1)

01.	Visitor:	How long were you married?
02.	Ms. Todd:	Uh we would've celebrated our- let's see.
03.		We- I think we celebrated our fiftieth anniversary
04.		and seemed like we're getting close to another one
05.		I don't know whether it was sixty or not
06.		but anyway we did celebrate our fiftieth.
07.	Visitor:	Oh that's awesome.
08.	Ms. Todd:	mmm hmm
09.	Visitor:	I hope to celebrate my fiftieth one day.
10.	Ms. Todd:	Yeah. That's about all I can tell you.
11.	Visitor:	Yeah, you have a lot of bells.
12.	Ms. Todd:	mmm hmm.
13.		I hadn't counted them.
14.		I should count 'em and see how [many (there are).
15.	Visitor:	[Well, let's count them and
16.		see how many there are.
17.	Ms. Todd:	You got time?
18.	Visitor:	Yeah!
19.	Ms. Todd:	You probably count faster than I do.
20.	Visitor:	Three, four, five, six, seven, eight, nine, ten, eleven, twelve,
21.		thirteen, fourteen, fifteen, sixteen, seventeen, eighteen,
22.		nineteen, twenty, twenty two, twenty three, twenty four, twenty five, twenty six
23.	Ms. Todd:	That's not bad at all [()
24.	Visitor:	[Twenty six bells. That's a lot of bells=
25.	Ms. Todd:	=It is.
26.	Visitor:	That's a fun thing to collect.

How does Ms. Todd respond initially (in lines 12–14) to the visitor's comment about the bells in line 11? What, then, does the visitor say to build on Ms. Todd's response? How might other responses by the visitor in lines 15–16 and line 18 have worked to advance or constrain this topic development?

Now review Extract 2c below which follows directly on the interaction represented in Extract 2b. Focus on the variety of ways in which both conversationalists talk about the bells. Turning first to the language used by the visitor, note the question posed in line 27 ("What made you collect bells?") and the memory gap that it uncovers in Ms. Todd (lines 28–32). How do the visitor and Ms. Todd then navigate the challenge of this memory gap? What other gaps in memory are displayed as the conversation unfolds and how are they managed?

Extract 2c: Bell collection (part 2)

27.	Visitor:	[What made you collect bells?
28.	Ms. Todd:	[(Uh huh) Uh seemed like somebody (.) gave me a bell
29.		and it just hit me in the head
30.		that I wanted to- collect them
31.		but I can't remember now who-
32.		I guess it was one of my grandchildren.
33.	Visitor:	'Cause of the pretty noise that it makes?
34.	Ms. Todd:	Well, that's, that's one thing.
35.		And I, I don't know,
36.		I just,
37.		it seems like somebody gave me some bells or a bell
38.		and I believe- yeah somebody brought me one from Hawaii.
39.		I believe that was one of my first ones.
40.	Visitor:	Oh [that's neat.
41.	Ms. Todd:	[And I like Mary and the baby too.
42.	Visitor:	Mmm hmm. (.)
43.		What about the one with the red roses on it
44.		that says love has a sound that hearts always hear?
45.	Ms. Todd:	Let's see if I can decide.
46.		I should have put the names who gave them to me.
47.		I can't remember now.
48.		I wish I [()
49.	Visitor:	[Maybe your husband gave you that one.
50.	Ms. Todd:	Uh I don't know.
51.	Visitor:	And that one's pretty too
52.		[the one with the hands?
53.	Ms. Todd:	[Mmm
54.		Mmm hmm.
55.	Visitor:	That's pretty.
56.	Ms. Todd:	The one with the little bear on top's cute too and Santa Claus.
57.	Visitor:	Mmm hmm
58.	Ms. Todd:	((*laughter*))
59.	Visitor:	That- that is cute,
60.		I like the bear.
61.	Ms. Todd:	I do too.
62.	Visitor:	Maybe I need to start collecting something.
63.	Ms. Todd:	Yeah. That's a good [idea.
64.	Visitor:	[You like that angel there.
65.		I like fairies.

66.	Ms. Todd:	Do you?
67.		Well collect- start collecting fairies
68.		and I'll buy you some
69.	Visitor:	They are just angelical aren't [they? they're just peaceful.=
70.	Ms. Todd:	[Mm hmm
71.		=They really are.
72.		So start collecting
73.		and I'll get you some.
74.	Visitor:	All right!
75.	Ms. Todd:	Yeah, we made those plates here, not too long ag- well,
76.		yeah it's been a good while
77.	Ms. Todd:	[( )
78.	Visitor:	[That plate's beautiful.
79.	Ms. Todd:	Isn't it pretty?

Throughout Extract 2c, what evidence can you find of agreement or disagreement between the speakers? How are these instances of (dis) agreement related to what they know or feel about the objects they're talking about? (Contrast, for example, lines 49–50 with lines 60–61.)

As the topic centered on the bell begins to wind down, consider how the visitor's utterance in line 62 shifts focus and opens up an opportunity for Ms. Todd to take more control and show a more agentive side (see especially lines 67–68 and 72–73). Note also how the conversationalists shift their joint attention away from the bells and on to new objects ("plates" in lines 75–79).

Activity 2b: You're the analyst

Comparing and contrasting conversations between guided art gallery tours and residential facilities

Now that you have read through ***Extracts 1a*** and ***1b*** (*photo calendar*), ***2a***, ***2b***, and ***2c*** (*bell collection*), and carried out the related activities, compare and contrast these interactions with those from the art gallery that were the focus of the first section of the chapter. What have you learned about the ways in which conversational partners can help or hinder meaningful engagement with persons with dementia?

Conclusion

Previous scholarly work has pointed to a proclivity for talk in the here-and-now by individuals with dementia. As noted above, examinations by Obler (1981) and Appell et al. (1982) provided early empirical evidence of what these scholars termed "context-" or "stimulus-boundedness." More recently, Bayles and Tomoeda (2014, pp. 229–231) have suggested that individuals with dementia "do best when the conversation concerns something they can see and feel, in other words, something to which they can refer." In specific connection to our study, they claim that a focus on physical objects may result in individuals with dementia "being able to call to mind other information that can be shared in the conversation."

These insights fit more generally into wider discussions by Snyder (2006), Basting (2006, 2009), and Kontos (2006) who recommend that individuals with dementia be given opportunities to engage in activities that downplay the focus on memory, since "self-esteem can be battered within therapies that focus on reminiscence or reality orientation, or even in personal interactions with family members and friends who insist on memory work" (Kontos, 2006). The challenge, then, is to devise activities that pivot away from a focus on memory, but still add value to one's life.

In this chapter, we witnessed individuals with dementia taking part in such activities by talking with others about physical objects in the here-and-now. In Section 1, we examined strategies employed by specially trained art gallery guides to create positive discourse environments that encouraged variegated verbal displays of lively minds as individuals with dementia and their companions engaged with works of art. In Section 2, we then explored dyadic conversations within assisted living apartments that included topics that were triggered by objects in clear view. While demonstrating some of the difficulties that may emerge as interlocutors attempt to maintain meaningful topics in the here-and-now, these interactions exemplified the caring philosophy expressed by Rust (1986) based on her conversations as a nursing assistant with individuals with dementia: "We sit and simply take up talking, wherever and whenever we are. Talking…is a wonderful experience in which we are always in the present, and *the present could be anything we choose to create between us.*"

These illustrations of "conversation as care" (Ryan, Byrne, Spykerman, & Orange, 2005) bring intentional focus—and offer a meaningful counterweight—to the overwhelming proportion of time typically spent in most assisted living, memory care, and skilled nursing facilities on "task-talk" (Backhaus, 2011, 2017; Williams & Warren, 2009). Along with the extracts from the art gallery examined above, they serve as a critical reminder of the important role environmental objects can play in nurturing meaningful interaction, especially when they are employed by attentive, compassionate, and creative conversational partners.

Practical Highlights

1. Conversations centered on objects that are present in the "here and now" may encourage persons with dementia to display their interests and knowledge.
2. Draw upon public objects (e.g., those in art museums or public spaces of care facilities) and private objects (e.g., personal photos, keepsakes) as potential topics of talk.
3. Allow, as much as possible, for the person with dementia to control the direction of the talk (e.g., they might initiate questions about the object, tell you something about it, or provide assessments in response to your own).
4. Look for opportunities to nurture meaningful interaction—be attentive, be compassionate, be creative.

Appendix

Transcription Conventions

(.)	pause in talk within a turn or lapse in talk between speaker turns
((*word*))	non-verbal behavior
<u>word</u>	emphasis
wo::rd	sound stretch
=	latched, or continuous talk
[ ]	overlapping talk
( )	inaudible talk
(word)	approximation of talk; transcriber uncertainty
°word°	talk that is spoken softly

Adapted from Goodwin, M. H. (1990). *He-said-she-said: Talk as social organization among Black children*. Bloomington, IN: Indiana University Press

References

Aaltonen, T., Arminen, I., & Raudaskoski, S. (2014). Photo sharing as a joint activity between an aphasic speaker and others. In M. Nevile, P. Haddington, T. Heinemann, & M. Rauniomaa (Eds.), *Interacting with objects: Language, materiality, and social activity* (pp. 125–144). Amsterdam, NL; Philadelphia, PA: John Benjamins.

Agar, M. (1985). Institutional discourse. *Text-Interdisciplinary Journal for the Study of Discourse, 5*(3), 147–168.

Ainsworth-Vaughn, N. (1998). *Claiming power in doctor-patient talk*. Oxford, UK: Oxford University Press.

Appell, J., Kertesz, A., & Fisman, M. (1982). A study of language functioning in Alzheimer patients. *Brain and Language, 17*(1), 73–91.

Backhaus, P. (Ed.). (2011). *Communication in elderly care: Cross-cultural perspectives*. London, UK: Bloomsbury Publishing.

Backhaus, P. (2017). *Care communication: Making a home in a Japanese eldercare facility*. New York, NY: Routledge.

Basting, A. D. (2006). Beyond the stigma of Alzheimer's. *Journal of Medical Humanities, 27*(2), 125–126.

Basting, A. D. (2009). *Forget memory: Creating better lives for people with dementia*. Baltimore, MD: The Johns Hopkins University Press.

Bayles, K., & Tomoeda, C. K. (2014). *Cognitive-communicative disorders of aging and dementia*. Boston, MA: Little, Brown and Company.

Bergmann, J. R. (1990). On the local sensitivity of conversation. In I. Markovà & K. Foppa (Eds.), *The dynamics of dialogue* (pp. 201–226). Hemel Hempstead, UK: Harvester Wheatsheaf.

Bolinger, D. (1957). *Interrogative structures of American English*. Birmingham, AL: University of Alabama Press.

Chafe, W. (1994). *Discourse, consciousness, and time: The flow and displacement of conscious experience in speaking and writing*. Chicago, IL: The University of Chicago Press.

Drew, P., & Heritage, J. (1992). Analyzing talk at work: An introduction. In P. Drew & J. Heritage (Eds.), *Talk at work: Interaction in institutional settings* (pp. 3–65). Cambridge, UK; New York, NY: Cambridge University Press.

Ford, C. (2010). Questioning in meetings: Participation and positioning. In A. Freed & S. Ehrlich (Eds.), *Why do you ask? The function of questions in institutional discourse* (pp. 211–234). Oxford, UK: Oxford University Press.

Freed, A. (2015). Institutional discourse. In K. Tracy, C. Ilie, & T. Sandel (Eds.), *The international encyclopedia of language & social interaction* (pp. 809–826). Boston, MA: Wiley.

Freed, A., & Ehrlich, S. (2010). *Why do you ask? The function of questions in institutional discourse*. Oxford, UK: Oxford University Press.

Garfinkel, H., & Wieder, L. D. (1992). Two incommensurable, asymmetrically alternate technologies of social analysis. In G. Watson & R. M. Seiler (Eds.), *Text in context: Contributions to ethnomethodology* (pp. 175–206). Newbury Park, CA: Sage.

Goodwin, C. (1994). Professional vision. *American Anthropologist, 96*(3), 606–633.

Goodwin, C. (2000). Action and embodiment within situated human interaction. *Journal of Pragmatics, 32*(10), 1489–1522.

Goodwin, C. (2013). The cooperative transformative organization of human action and knowledge. *Journal of Pragmatics, 46*(1), 8–23.

Goodwin, C. (2017). *Co-operative action*. Cambridge, UK; New York, NY: Cambridge University Press.

Hamilton, H. E. (2008). Narrative as snapshot: Glimpses into the past in Alzheimer's discourse. *Narrative Inquiry, 18*(1), 53–82.

Hamilton, H. E. (2011). At the intersection of art, Alzheimer's disease, and discourse: Talk in the surround of paintings. In P. Backhaus (Ed.), *Communication in elderly care: Cross-cultural approaches* (pp. 166–193). London, UK: Continuum.

Hamilton, H. E. (2019). *Language, dementia and meaning making: Navigating challenges of cognition and face in everyday life*. London, UK: Palgrave Macmillan.

Heritage, J. (1984). A change-of state token and aspects of its sequential placement. In J. M. Atkinson & J. Heritage (Eds.), *Structure of social action: Studies in conversation analysis* (pp. 299–345). Cambridge, UK: Cambridge University Press.

Heritage, J. (2004). Conversation analysis and institutional talk. In K. L. Fitch & R. E. Sanders (Eds.), *Handbook of language and social interaction* (pp. 103–147). Mahwah, NJ: Lawrence Erlbaum Associates.

Heritage, J. (2012). Epistemics in action: Action formation and territories of knowledge. *Discourse Studies, 45*(1), 1–29.

Heritage, J., & Clayman, S. (2010). *Talk in action: Interactions, identities, and institutions*. Oxford, UK: Wiley-Blackwell.

Heritage, J., & Raymond, G. (2005). The terms of agreement: Indexing epistemic authority and subordination in talk-in-interaction. *Social Psychology Quarterly, 68*(1), 15–38.

Hodges, J. R. (2000). Memory in the dementias. In E. Tulving & F. I. M. Craik (Eds.), *The Oxford handbook of memory* (pp. 441–464). New York, NY: Oxford University Press.

Housen, A. (1999). Eye of the beholder: Research, theory and practice. Paper presented at the conference of "Aesthetic and art education: A transdisciplinary approach" sponsored by the Calouste Gulbenkian Foundation, Service of Education, September 27–29, 1999, Lisbon, PT.

Hultgren, A. K., & Cameron, D. (2010). 'How may I help you?': Questions, control, and customer care in telephone call center talk. In A. Freed & S. Ehrlich (Eds.), *Why do you ask? The function of questions in institutional discourse* (pp. 322–342). Oxford, UK: Oxford University Press.

Kesner, R. P., & Hunsaker, M. R. (2010). The temporal attributes of episodic memory. *Behavioural Brain Research, 215*(2), 299–309.

Kontos, P. C. (2006). Embodied selfhood: An ethnographic exploration of Alzheimer's disease. In A. Leibing & L. Cohen (Eds.), *Thinking about dementia: Culture, loss, and the anthropology of senility* (pp. 195–217). New Brunswick, NJ: Rutgers University Press.

MacPherson, S., Bird, M., Anderson, K., Davis, T., & Blair, A. (2009). An art gallery access programme for people with dementia: "You do it for the moment". *Aging & Mental Health, 13*(5), 744–752.

Nevile, M., Haddington, P., Heinemann, T., & Rauniomaa, M. (2014). On the interactional ecology of objects. In M. Nevile, P. Haddington, T. Heinemann, & M. Rauniomaa (Eds.), *Interacting with objects: Language, materiality, and social activity* (pp. 3–26). Amsterdam, NL; Philadelphia, PA: John Benjamins.

Obler, L. (1981). Review of Le langage des déments by Luce Irigaray. *Brain and Language, 12*(2), 375–386.
Pope, C., & Davis, B. H. (2011). Finding a balance: The Carolinas Conversation Collection. *Corpus Linguistics and Linguistic Theory, 7*(1), 143–161.
Ritchhart, R. (2007). Cultivating a culture of thinking in museums. *Journal of Museum Education, 32*(2), 137–152.
Rust, L. (1986). Another part of the country. In J. Alexander, D. Berrow, L. Domitrovich, M. Donnelly, & C. McLean (Eds.), *Women and aging: An anthology by women* (pp. 137–147). Corvallis, OR: Calyx Books.
Ryan, E. B., Byrne, K., Spykerman, H., & Orange, J. B. (2005). Evidencing Kitwood's personhood strategies: Conversation as care in dementia. In B. H. Davis (Ed.), *Alzheimer talk, text and context: Enhancing communication* (pp. 190–198). New York, NY: Palgrave Macmillan.
Searle, J. R. (1969). *Speech acts: An essay in the philosophy of language.* Cambridge, UK: Cambridge University Press.
Schegloff, E. A. (2007). *Sequence organization in interaction: A primer in conversation analysis.* Cambridge, UK; New York, NY: Cambridge University Press.
Shelley-Tremblay, J. (2011). The breakdown of semantics in aphasia and dementia. In J. Guendouzi, F. Loncke, & M. J. Williams (Eds.), *The handbook of psycholinguistic and cognitive processes* (pp. 625–645). New York, NY: Psychology Press.
Sidnell, J. (2015). Epistemics. In K. Tracy (Ed.), *The international encyclopedia of language and social interaction* (pp. 1–13). Hoboken, NJ: Wiley.
Snyder, L. (2006). Personhood and interpersonal communication in dementia. In J. C. Hughes, S. J. Louw, & S. R. Sabat (Eds.), *Dementia: Mind, meaning and the person* (pp. 259–276). Oxford, UK: Oxford University Press.
Stivers, T., Mondada, L., & Steensig, J. (2011). Knowledge, morality and affiliation in social interaction. In T. Stivers, L. Mondada, & J. Steensig (Eds.), *The morality of knowledge in conversation* (pp. 3–24). Cambridge, UK: Cambridge University Press.
Streeck, J., Goodwin, C., & LeBaron, C. (2011). *Embodied interaction: Language and body in the material world.* Cambridge, UK: Cambridge University Press.
vom Lehn, D., Heath, C., & Hindmarsh, J. (2005). Examining exhibits: Interaction in museums and galleries. *Communication and Cognition Monographies, 38*(3–4), 229–247.

Williams, K. N., & Warren, C. A. (2009). Communication in assisted living. *Journal of Aging Studies, 23*(1), 24–36.
Zeisel, J. (2009). *I'm still here: A breakthrough approach to understanding someone living with Alzheimer's*. New York, NY: Penguin Group.

Recommended Readings

Backhaus, P. (2017b). *Care communication: Making a home in a Japanese eldercare facility*. New York, NY: Routledge.
Basting, A. D. (2009). *Forget memory: Creating better lives for people with dementia*. Baltimore, MD: The Johns Hopkins University Press.
Davis, B. H. (Ed.). (2005). *Alzheimer talk, text and context: Enhancing communication*. New York, NY: Palgrave Macmillan.
Hamilton, H. E. (2019). *Language, dementia and meaning making: Navigating challenges of cognition and face in everyday life*. London, UK: Palgrave Macmillan.
Hughes, J. C., Louw, S. J., & Sabat, S. R. (Eds.). (2005). *Dementia: Mind, meaning and the person*. Oxford, UK: Oxford University Press.
Leibing, A., & Cohen, L. (Eds.). (2006). *Thinking about dementia: Culture, loss, and the anthropology of senility*. New Brunswick, NJ: Rutgers University Press.
Nevile, M., Haddington, P., Heinemann, T., & Rauniomaa, M. (Eds.). (2014). *Interacting with objects: Language, materiality, and social activity*. Amsterdam, NL; Philadelphia, PA: John Benjamins.
Streeck, J., Goodwin, C., & LeBaron, C. (2011). *Embodied interaction: Language and body in the material world*. Cambridge, UK: Cambridge University Press.

9

Disagreements in Assessment Sequences with Persons Diagnosed with Frontotemporal Dementia

Michael Sean Smith

Learning Objectives

By the end of this chapter, you will be able to:

- Identify assessment sequences and the social import of atypical second assessments in persons with frontotemporal (and possibly other) dementia;
- Realign conversational expectations for such anomalies in order to circumvent disruptions in social actions such as collaborative meaning-making—intersubjectivity—and/or establishment of epistemic relationships.

This chapter examines how assessment sequences prove to be difficult within the conversations of a person diagnosed with frontotemporal dementia (FTD). *Assessments*, or the expression of valued statements

M. S. Smith (✉)
Linköping University, Linköping, Sweden
e-mail: michael.smith@liu.se

T. Stickle (ed.), *Learning from the Talk of Persons with Dementia*,
The Language of Mental Health, https://doi.org/10.1007/978-3-030-43977-4_9

have been documented within mundane conversations between neurotypical or unimpaired co-participants as a means to affective and experiential collaboration between participants (Goodwin, 1980; Goodwin & Goodwin, 1987). In this way, assessments in mundane conversations work to develop shared understanding, i.e., *intersubjectivity*, and build relationships. Assessments have also been shown as a way by which the negotiation of epistemic authority and subordination between participants are established, maintained, and changed (Heritage & Raymond, 2005; Raymond & Heritage, 2006). As FTD is a neuropathological syndrome that disrupts social behavior impacting both intersubjective co-construction in activities and alignment in interpersonal relationships, the employment of assessments within conversations with persons with FTD is examined within this chapter. Here, analyses of assessment activities between a female FTD patient and her co-participants show that inabilities to provide such secondary assessment utterances in sequential and turn placement along with other disruptions does, indeed, negatively affect the collaborations of meaning, the development of interpersonal relationships, and the negotiation of epistemic alignments for the participants within these conversations. Awareness of potential difficulties in conversation with participants diagnosed with FTD may provide co-participants better expectations *of* and preparedness *fo*r displays that lie outside the norm in such conversations.

Introduction

Frontotemporal Dementia

Frontotemporal dementia is a degenerative dementia that causes neural atrophy in the frontal lobes and the anterior temporal lobes (Snowden, Neary, & Mann, 2002). Several variants of FTD exist and are differentiated by regional and/or hemispherical distribution of the atrophy (Feldman & Kertesz, 2001; Kertesz, 2003; Mesulam, 2001; Rosen et al., 2002).

This chapter will concentrate on the behavioral disturbances associated with FTD with asymmetrical involvement in the right frontal and/or anterior temporal lobes. The current consensus defines several behavioral features of FTD to include the decline in social conduct, emotional blunting, impairment in regulating personal conduct, as in becoming too passive or overactive, and having impaired insight. The social and emotional disturbances so predominate in FTD of the right hemisphere is a result of the importance that this neurological area plays in regulating social interaction and emotional regulation, and thus the further study of FTD is important in understanding the neurological processes involved in these areas.

Assessments

Assessments are conversational actions that participants produce in interaction in which one individual constructs an utterance either with one or more parts—technically Turn Constructional Units (TCU)—that contains both a referent (the assessable) and the actual assessment, or value statement, of that assessable. Assessments may be positive or negative or somewhere in between. After the first assessment, other participants must decide how they want to treat the first assessment. Pomerantz defined "second assessments" as "assessments produced by recipients of prior assessments in which the referents in the seconds are the same as those in the first" (Pomerantz, 1984, p. 59).

Assessments first rely on the participants' *joint attention* to specific environmental or ideational artifacts. That is, a participant employs an assessment of something within the shared purview—physical or abstract—of the participants engaged within the conversation. When a first assessment is employed, then "a relevant action for a co-participant is to agree or disagree with the assessment offered in the prior turn" (Ogden, 2005, p. 1754): this is referred to as a second assessment. As it turns out, whether producers of the second assessments wish to produce strong or weak dis/agreements is related to and revealed by the timing and lexical choices of their assessment (Pomerantz, 1984). The timing and lexical choices of participants in producing assessment activities is connected to the general preference structures found in adjacency pairs;

with preference here being the "normative organization, where deviations from the norm are accountable by and/or problematic for participants" (Ogden, 2005, p. 1755). In short, first position positive and negative assessments prefer, in both valence and strength, to be followed by a second position assessment, and any deviation from this highlights differences in position between participants around the same referent or assessable and could possibly lead to dis-alignment or even conflict. For example, if a participant makes a first assessment, what has been shown to be the normative response by a co-participant is a second assessment:

First assessment A: The room is decorated lovely.
Second assessment B: Yes, the colors are very warm and relaxing.

We may easily envision how important assessment activities are, then, in the negotiation of mutual alignment or dis-alignment in interaction. Goffman first pointed out that "by saying something, the speaker opens himself up to the possibility that the intended recipients will…think him forward, foolish, or offensive in what he has said" (1967, p. 37). Assessments doubly emphasize this possibility since speakers bring into play assessables and their specific positive or negative assessments toward them. This is highlighted in Charles and Marjorie Goodwin's study of the concurrent organization of assessments, where they noted "in assessing something of being a specific value, the speaker publicly commits himself to that evaluation of that object. Then recipients, by its public display, can then judge both the assessed item and the speaker by making the assessment" (1987, p. 9). Furthermore, assessments as an activity provide a place for participants to display not only their stance toward the immediately occurring talk but to the experiential and affective stance taken toward that object or experience; so much often that "the apparent referent of the assessment becomes far less important than the shared affect and co-experience the participants display to each other" (Goodwin & Goodwin, 1987, p. 41). So, an inherent aspect of assessments is in their occasioned opportunity for individuals to affectively and experientially bond in talk. Communion, however, is not the only property of assessments but can also be grounds for differentiation. Heritage and Raymond have shown that in many situations, assessments can also be used for asserting exclusive or singular epistemic or relational rights to specific forms of knowledge. In this they noted that while "affiliation and agreement generally are sought from others; when provided, however, they must respect the parties' information territories and their associated epistemic rights" (Heritage & Raymond, 2005, p. 36). Assessments activities, in both their explicit production and in their implicit or underlying biases, present an excellent opportunity for participants to coordinate the intersubjective grounds for both communion and separation in interaction and, thereby, foster a better relationship.

Thinking Point

Imagine yourself offering a positive assessment of a painting in the room you and a friend are occupying:
A: What a beautiful landscape.
Now, your co-participant might issue a second assessment that agrees:
B: Yes, it is lovely. It reminds me of my childhood home.
Or, the co-participant could issue a second assessment that does not agree:

B: Agh, that painting is hideous. Who on earth paid money for that!
The negotiation of assessments has the potential to build or stress relationships.

Data and Methods

The current analysis is based on an observation of an FTD patient Freda, aged 72, who exhibits the right frontal and temporal variant of the disease. The patient and family were visited twice for four hours each visit. The researcher interacted with and observed the patients interacting with family members in everyday settings, with each visit audio and videotaped. The video and audio records were transcribed and examined using the orthography and precepts of conversational analysis (CA) as described by Sacks, Schegloff, and Jefferson (1974).

The main precept of this chapter is that—given the importance of assessment activities in the maintenance of social relations in interaction and given the profound social disturbances that FTD patients suffer in social conduct and intersubjective collaboration—it might be beneficial to look at assessment sequences in interaction with FTD patients for what they can tell us about the interactional difficulties that can arise within their relationships.

Analysis

Now, the analysis presented below and the subsequent arguments made from it should be qualified. It is comprised of a small corpus of data (about eight hours for the one patient) and the examples provided represent an undefined subset of this corpus. The arguments made then should not be seen as definitive but rather initial in their orientation. The purpose of this analysis is then just an explorative foray into looking at well-studied findings in the conversational/interactional analytic tradition and looking at how the presence of this dementia has an influence on these features of social interaction. This initial view may help to inform caregivers, family, and practitioners on how assessments and second assessments may be addressed by persons with FTD and help co-participants manage their expectations of such interactions.

Second Assessments in the Talk of a Person with FTD

In the context of this first extract, the patient, Freda, and her caregiver are looking through a novelty and collectible shop near the patient's house. In this specific extract, Penny has just looked to something and called Freda's attention to it, through a summons, a directive, and then finally an assessment to the assessable: "flowers."

Extract 1: "Gardenias"

```
01.   Penny:    Freda
02.   Freda:    Yes
03.   Penny:    Freda^ >look at these<beautiful flow^ers
04.             in this little [(0.6) they're gardenias
05.   Freda:                   [Yeah^, I kno:w^
06.             but what I want to do is-
07.             that [it's my wonder of=
08.   Penny:         [°Yea(h)h. ((turned away from
                      Freda))
09.             =the world I want to go
10.             down and cross and go back
11.   Penny:    Okay? ((turned towards Freda))
12.   Freda:    Okay?
13.   Penny:    Yeah,
```

Essential before looking at the actual turn construction of Freda's turn in lines 04–06, and 08–09 (the appropriate place for the second assessment), it is important to first examine how Penny orients toward the sequence from its beginning. In lines 01, 03, and 04, we see Penny produces a summons (an address), a directive (an imperative for action on the part of the co-participant), and then a final pre-positioned assessment, "beautiful" to the assessable, "flowers" (Goodwin & Goodwin, 1987). Forgoing intensive scrutiny of Freda's turn, we can see that Penny's production in line 08, during Freda's ongoing turn, constitutes a continuer of sorts. Charles Goodwin (1986) from Schegloff (1992) described continuers as utterances that display that the hearers' understanding of the preceding talk—a multi-TCU (part) turn—is in progress but not complete. The continuer also collaborates in the achievement of that multi-TCU utterance "by passing the opportunity to either (a) produce a more extended turn of their own or (b) initiate repair on the talk just heard" (1986, p. 207).The continuer, thus, functions as a "bridge" between two TCUs of a multi-TCU turn. Here, however, we see something a little different is being produced by Penny. Penny's apparent continuer does not come in at an orderly place of speaker change, i.e., a transition relevant place (TRP). Instead, Penny launches her next turn of talk at a point where Freda's turn is not possibly complete:

Extract 1A: "Gardenias"

05.	Freda:	[Yeah^, I kno:w^
06.		but what I want to do is-
07.		that [it's my wonder of=
08.	Penny:	[°Yea(h)h. *((turned away from Freda))*
09.	Freda:	=the world I want to go
10.		down and cross and go back

Qualitatively, in Penny's turn in line 08, there is certain "defeatedness" in its prosodic quality. It is produced in a silent manner, consisting mostly of aspiration, or breathiness, rather than voicing, and finalizes with a downward intonation. In concordance with this, Penny has actually turned away both during her production, which overlaps Freda's turn, and before the completion of Freda's ongoing turn. Penny's turn is, thus, not displaying embodied reception of Freda's turn. Its placement and production, then, suggests that its affective referent is more of what the patient has done (or not done) than what the patient is about to do. And given its affective downgrade, it seems to signal that Freda has in some way not completed the expected action that she was selected for by Penny's prior turn in lines 03 and 04. Penny does not come around to produce voiced and embodied turns (in lines 11 and 13) until after Freda's productions in lines 09, 10, and 12, which are actually just reformulations of Freda's desired next action (which is to leave the store and continue on their routine back to her home). It is at line 11 that Penny turns toward and gives visual receipt of Freda's declarative turn. So, just from this presentation of the data above, we could say that while the patient does perform in some manner that is pragmatically/ appropriate, that is, answering to the summons, by placing a response after Penny's assessment, Freda does not, however, respond to Penny's assessment in a typical, expected manner. Penny seems to also mark this ill-treatment by her own response. In essence, Penny's subsequent talk affirms this as it does not treat Freda's utterance as a second assessment.

If we turn, however, to the actual construction of Freda's turn, it becomes a little more complicated. (I have omitted line 8, which contained Penny's utterance.)

Extract 1B: "Gardenias"

05.	Freda:	[Yeah^, I kno:w^
06.		but what I want to do is-
07.		that [it's my wonder of=
09.		=the world I want to go
10.		down and cross and go back

Freda's multipart turn begins with "Yeah, I know." In this TCU, Freda begins with a displayed affective, emotion-filled, utterance toward Penny's prior assessment, but then quickly segues into another TCU beginning with "but," a contrastive lexical construct. What this seems to do is treat Penny's prior assessment as a "knowable" and without giving additional treatment as to its validity. Hence, Freda does not provide a second assessment but rather treats Penny's assessment as unnecessary for reciprocal or contrary assessment. What Freda does, instead, is to contrast Penny's assessment with something that is more desirable or interactionally important, thus socially diminishing Penny's prior assessment. This then sheds light on Penny's defeated and non-aligned production of the subsequent continuer (Extract 1A, line 08).

Freda suddenly self-repairs (i.e., self corrects) her action and moves into what is actually a positive assessment: "it's my wonder of the world." "Wonder of the world" was a repetitive assessment that Freda used in many different situations. This, however, was not just a rote expression unresponsive in its deployment. The two examples below show the assessment to be adequately sensitive to its environmental production.

Extract 2: Wonder of the World
((Penny is talking to Diane; Freda is talking to both Penny and Diane))

04.	Penny:	The lady down here at (this) place
05.	Freda:	I used to sell at everything
06.	-->	I was a wonder of [the world=
07	Diane:	[I've never been down there=
08.	Freda:	=and I've known her for years and years
09.	Diane:	=(xxxx)

Extract 3: Wonder of the World (2)

((Penny is talking to a stranger couple in a novelty shop))

05.	Freda:	You wanna know something? ((*To Man/Couple*))
06.	Freda:	The people down there got this one here
07.	------>	and it is a<wonder of the world>.

In these two examples, we see Freda using her "wonder of the world" assessment. Her production in both instances and other instances shows it to alter, according to the context of production, in its syntactic, lexical, and referential construction. While it may not semantically fit, Freda's assessment is sensitive to the physical and social environment in which it is spoken, and is interpretable by others in such a way. In the "Gardenias" extract, however, Penny does not give receipt of the turn and in looking at the construction of Freda's turn, we can see this to be a result of the conflict between the turn's sequential placement, the action this placement requires, and the assessment's placement within the turn:

Extract 1B: "Gardenias"

05.	Freda:	[Yeah^, I kno:w^
06.		but what I want to do is-
07.	----->	that [it's my wonder of=
09.	----->	=the world I want to go
10.		down and cross and go back

If we look at Freda's turn (05), we can see first the affirmation receipt "Yeah, I know," then we see the beginning of the next TCU at "but what I want to do is-,." The second assessment comes to form a type of declarative proposal, specifically her desire to leave the store and continue on her routine. Simply put, Freda's turn, regardless of its construction, should display first an adequate treatment of the prior turn, action, or context and a fully interpretable "interactional track" for what should come next—what Schegloff (1992, pp. 1315–1316) has called "second order organization." The initial position and the final position of the relevant TCUs and their ordering becomes the most crucial aspect, since these are the "exchange points" for the intersubjective (collaborative meaning-making) to occur. We can see some of the underlying mechanisms of Freda's turn and, from the anomalies to mundane conversation order, some of the reasons why Penny did not receive it. Though it appears that Freda's turn contains three actions: (1) the affirmation, (2) the proposed next action with the (3) parenthetical assessment, interactionally the turn has two actions: the assessment and the proposed next action.

We can see the transformation of Freda's use of 'it's my wonder of the world' here:

Extract 1B: "Gardenias"

05.	Freda:	[Yeah^, I kno:w^
06.		but what I want to do is-
07.		that [it's my wonder of=
09.		=the world I want to go
10.		down and cross and go back

to this: `Freda:` `Yeah, I know that` <u>`it's my wonder of the world`</u> `but what I want to do is I want to go down and cross and go back.`

While transformation is partially speculative, there is evidence for it in Freda's turn. First, the presence of Freda's assessment but also her demonstrative "reordering" of the turn depicts the underlined utterance's transformability—at least this one that we have seen Freda, at various times, use as different actions. At her "but what I want to do is-," (Extract 1B, line 06) Freda suddenly cuts off her own production (line 07) and inserts something she displays as belonging earlier: the assessment. Here then, Freda's initial "Yeah, I know" becomes less dismissive in its affection and more affirmative. In this we see, much like "normal" individuals, the speaker "can interrupt components-in-progress in order to insert ones that 'belong' earlier" (Schegloff, 1992, pp. 1315–1316), so as to be receptive to others' prior actions. But unlike other "normal" individuals, there appears to a lack of orientation to the necessity of the ordering for the benefit of others. This conflict in ordering presents not only in the balancing between the other speaker's prior turn and next turn in attempts at aligning assessments, but can become especially acute in assessment activities where the patient is demonstratively constructing a dispreferred assessment to the prior one.

Thinking Points

- When co-participants do not produce the next actions we expect, trouble in our social relationships can emerge.
- When persons diagnosed with dementia do not produce the next actions we expect, giving pause to contemplate how their next turns maybe, indeed, affected by their condition, maybe enough to ward off our normal troubled reactions.

In this next extract "It's Broken" Freda, her friend Diane, and Penny, her caretaker, are shopping in another collectible store. Diane, Freda's friend, finds something and is trying to get Freda to reciprocate an assessment toward it.

Extract 4: It's Broken

Diane:	(xxxx) Isn't this darling *((Diane*
	holding object;
Penny:	I love it
Diane:	Freda this is so cute *((Freda walks to Diane))*
Penny:	Freda you should get that
Penny:	[Its-
Freda:	[No I don't like it.
Penny:	No she [doesn't like it.]
Diane:	[I:: li:ke i::t]
Freda:	Really [No.
Diane:	[I like it (a lot)
Freda:	No because this one's broken (.) here
	((*pointing to object*))
Diane:	[Oh
Freda:	[This is broke here *((Then starts to turn*
	around and move away))
Diane:	Ohh [It's broken *((Mouthing to Penny))*
Penny:	[*((Penny starts laughing))*
Freda:	It's Broken *((Walking out of the*
	store))
Diane:	Mm mh
Penny:	Hih hheh heh heh No [take it back heh
	((Penny in play voice))
?????	[(xxxxx)
Penny:	No take it back heh heh *((Diane and*
	Penny follow Freda out of store))

Up until Freda's assessment in line 07, we see both of the other participants constructing positive assessments toward the object. Diane is the first to assess the object holding it up for both Penny and Freda in lines 01 and 02. At this point, Penny commits to an upgraded self-referential second assessment in line 03 during which Freda walks toward Diane holding the object. As Freda is moving toward Diane, Diane produces another like-assessment in line 04, at which point Penny then produces her supportive recommend: "Freda you should get that." Freda here then produces her assessment, "No I don't like it." It is unclear whether Freda's utterance is a second assessment to Diane's and Penny's original assessments or whether it is just responsive to Penny's prior turn in line 05, but, regardless, by this point, both Diane and Penny have made several "commitments" to their assessments, and as a result, require validation or treatment interactionally by their placement. This is especially true since Diane's and Penny's "commitments" to the assessable were especially strong or upgraded, with Diane's negative interrogative in line 01 and Penny's declarative "I love it."

Extract 4A: "It's broken"

07.	Freda:	[No I don't like it.
08.	Penny:	No she [doesn't like it.]
09.	Diane:	[I:: li:ke i::t]
		((To Freda))
10.	Freda:	Really [No.
11.	Diane:	[I like it (a lot)
		((To Freda))

How first assessments, especially those that are intensely upgraded, commit their speaker's in interaction is evident in Diane's turns in lines 09 and 11. While Penny essentially drops the interactional track after Freda's assessment, Diane continues by first producing a turn in line 09 that explicates the affective and experiential reasoning behind her first assessment in the simplest terms in line 01. When this again does not provide for a reciprocal assessment from Freda, Diane explicitly recycles her prior utterance in line 11 with a possible upgrade. In these actions, we can see that in the face of adverse uptake of Diane's assessment, she continuously moves to defend its position. This trend continues in the interaction, though in the next turn, Freda produces something that is significant:

Extract 4B: "It's Broken"

Diane:	[I like it (a lot)
Freda:	No because this one's broken (.) here
	((pointing to object))
Diane:	[Oh
Freda:	[This is broke here *((Then starts to turn*
	around and move away))
Diane:	Ohh [It's broken *((Mouthing to Penny))*
Penny:	[*((Penny starts laughing))*
Freda:	It's Broken *((Walking out of the*
	store))
Diane:	Mm mh
Penny:	Hih hheh heh heh No [take it back heh
	((Penny in play voice))
?????	[(xxxxx)
Penny:	No take it back heh heh *((Diane and*
	Penny follow Freda out of store))

At line 12, Freda then moves to point out that the object that Diane was holding was "broken" pointing to a part of the object (which appeared to be a practical or ornamental hummingbird feeder). Now, while Diane initially gives receipt of Freda's reasoning, she quickly displays to Penny in a silent mocking fashion that the feeder is indeed not broken. To which Penny begins laughing and then starts to mock-affirm Freda's reasoning by mock-telling Diane to "take it back," all while producing laugh tokens.

While something could probably be said that Freda produces an incorrect version of reality (at least according to the other participants) in her reasoning, what is significant for this analysis of assessment activities with the patient is that in this placement, she produces an "account" for her dispreferred assessment. This is important because in doing dispreferred turns, participants often produce accounts so as to mitigate the potential social fallout from doing dis-aligned actions by giving a reason for their necessity (Schegloff, 2007, p. 65), and so Freda's second assessment and its subsequent "accounting" do not seem out of variance with past research on assessment activities. So again, we see that like in the last extract, what seems to be at issue for the patient and her co-participants is not the absence of the produced action, but rather its specific ordering or placement, vis-à-vis others' actions. The problem seems not in the absence of producing a socially desired or relevant action (though this does occur, especially when the patient's attention has not been secured) but rather in its ordering from or toward others' actions. The problem then may not be in the patient interactionally orientating toward specific actions that must be completed (second assessments to firsts; accounts given after dispreferred actions) but rather in utilizing the minute and acute interactional space that is delineated for these actions to take place.

This problematic use of interactional space between and within turns at talk may be something that is implicitly managed by the other participants in interaction. The extract given below is indicative of this. Here Freda, Diane, and Penny are walking along the storefronts when Freda turns to Diane and initiates the following exchange:

Extract 5: "fifteen dollars or less"

Freda:	I want to show you something (.)
	that's only<fifteen years old> (xx)
	(0.8)
Diane:	Oh
Penny:	Fifteen dollars or less
Freda:	Fifteen dollars [or less
Diane:	[Oh that place is great(.).
	isn't it?
Freda:	Yes= *((nods to Diane))*
Diane:	=I know the one you're talking about…
	((continued…))

In the extract above, while there is an interesting phenomenon in priming on the subjects semantic construction (just prior to this exchange, the two other participants were talking about relationships that spanned years and "years older" was used by Diane), for the purposes of this current analysis, we see three relevant features to the successful production of assessment activities in interactions with the patient. First the co-participant, Diane, moves to produce the first assessment within a context where the patient has already committed herself to a topical initiation and continuance. This provides for maximal probability that when the assessment is produced, the patient will be already oriented toward its referent with little expenditure on reorientation. Also, since the patient has already committed to an expected evaluation of the referent, Diane is able to produce a like-assessment in the first position. Second, in producing the first assessment, Diane in line 07 first produces a simple declarative assessment but then after a micro-pause tag a negative interrogative at the end, highly biasing Freda's response for a yes, reducing the second assessment down to its most basic form: simple affirmation. Third and finally, Diane then moves to circumscribe the interactional space to which Freda has responded "yes" in constructing her second assessment, by quickly producing an additional TCU in line 10. What is interesting is that Diane moves to provide the referential material for Freda with "I know the one you're talking about..." thereby filling in the content that may or may have not been in Freda's possible second assessment. Other possible ways to help the patient produce an assessment include (1) waiting for the patient to be engaged in the referential content or (2) choosing a referent that one could expect the patient to be highly motivated to speak about.

Thinking Points

Two strategies emerged in the data that may help persons with dementia orient and respond in more typical ways:

- Prime the person for the first assessment by, for instance, picking up or pointing to an object before commenting on it;
- Ensure the person shares or is engaged in the same reference (physical or abstract) of the ongoing conversation.

Example: Pick up a photograph, point to it, ensure the patient sees your engagement with the photograph, and then issue an assessment, such as 'This child is pretty.' If there is no response and the person with dementia still seems to pay attention, issue an upgraded assessment, for instance, 'she is really is very beautiful.' Give the person time to respond.

Summary

The analysis presented above presents a highly complicated view of some of the behavioral problems evident in FTD, and there really are no straightforward conclusions that can be easily drawn from the analysis. It is evident, if not readily definable, that persons with FTD, and perhaps with other types of dementia as well, have trouble in assessment activities and that these troubles have serious consequences for how such persons are perceived socially, clinically, and culturally. The patient Freda is socially seen by others as not orienting toward either her interlocutors or to the interactional activities that they are trying to engage her in. Because the strategies employed involve activities that comprise some of the most basic actions that participants use to establish understanding and build interpersonal relationships, the trouble displayed in the extracts show disruptions in such common human activities as affective attunement, social bonding, self-differentiation. As a result, Freda, or others who display similar problems, is seen as being emotionally distant, self-centered, or emotionally disinhibited. When we look, however, at patients' actual conduct in interaction and how they construct their actions, and we compare these to well-studied activities in interaction with non-impaired individuals, then we see that it seems that the inability to supply expected interactional actions, such as second assessments, can impair relationships with even the closest co-participants: family members, caregivers, clinicians, or other practitioners. A simple orientation to these interactional anomalies, then, may help alleviate the unintended, but nevertheless, negative effect, which is producing misalignment, dis-alignment, conflict.

In mundane conversations between unimpaired participants, there seems to be an acute interactional space both in between and within turns that requires certain actions for understanding and relationship building. The consequences for the absence of such actions are apparent in the extracts above. In the first extract, Penny did not produce receipt of the second assessment because its presence was hidden by its placement within the turn. Because Freda did not produce her account early enough, Diane acted to produce two additional explicit reformulations of her prior assessment, whereby she had to reaffirm her commitment to the assessable, which was then never reciprocated. In these extracts, the patient's orientation toward necessary social productions was either completely invisible or too late in their production. This analysis shows how fine-tuned the coordination of assessment productions needs to be in order to initiate and substantiate the affective and social benefits.

What is also apparent is how ingrained these expectations are for us that the presence of a diagnosis that sufficiently accounts for the action(s) absence is not sufficient for the co-participant to give an immediate or automatic pass for the anomalies in the talk. This is perhaps the crux of this chapter: being prepared for such anomalies may, in fact, assuage the non-impaired participant of any negative assessment or interactional obligations felt toward the person with dementia.

The last extract may show some of the biases that are inherent in FTD, and how these relate to the problematic production of assessment activities in interactions with the patients. What seems to be of crucial importance for successful first and second assessment activities with the patients is either to take opportunity of the patient's already displayed engagement with possible assessables, and then produce the first assessment so as to highly circumscribe the type of assessment that the patient can make and the spatial extent to which they have to make the assessment. Or, the patient's co-participants can again take opportunity of the already present engagement, and select the patient for first assessment through a simple "noticing." In both cases though, we see that the patient's co-participants must actively work to first establish the probable prediction of the patient's intersubjective position so as to design the assessments or noticings to maximize for reciprocal or initial attempt at alignment. What may be a difficulty then for the patients in other scenarios is in the online reorientation toward the intersubjective, or shared, position of others in interaction so as to produce socially appropriate actions not for the sake of their own existence but for the sake of the co-participants' necessities who require those actions in specific points in time and space. Positioning the actions of talk so that participants with dementia can respond accordingly is, perhaps, the best way to ensure they may demonstrate retained competencies within such mundane interactions and prevent disruptions in interpersonal relationships.

Practical Highlights

1. Anomalies in common conversational actions, such as providing expected secondary assessments, may occur within interactions with persons diagnosed with FTD or other dementias.
2. Being prepared for these anomalies may mitigate social trouble such as viewing the person with dementia as interactionally or socially incompetent.
3. Strategies such as priming or ensuring the person with dementia is oriented to a shared interactional topic (e.g., physical or otherwise), may also engender better and more socially conducive conversations.

References

Feldman, H., & Kertesz, A. (2001). Diagnosis, classification and natural history of degenerative dementias. *Canadian Journal of Neurological Sciences, 28*(1), S17–S27.

Goffman, E. (1967). *Interaction ritual: Essays in face to face behavior*. Garden City, NY: Doubleday.

Goodwin, C. (1986). Between and within: Alternative sequential treatments of continuers and assessments. *Human Studies, 9,* 205–217.

Goodwin, M. H. (1980). Processes of mutual monitoring implicated in the production of description sequences. *Sociological Inquiry, 50*(3–4), 303–317.

Goodwin, M. H., & Goodwin, C. (1987). Concurrent operations on talk: Notes on the interactive organization of assessments. *IPrA Papers in Pragmatics, 1,* 1–55.

Heritage, J., & Raymond, G. (2005). The terms of agreement: Indexing epistemic authority and subordination in assessment sequences. *Social Psychology Quarterly, 65,* 15–38.

Kertesz, A. (2003). Pick complex: An integrative approach to frontotemporal dementia—Primary progressive aphasia, corticobasal degeneration, and progressive supranuclear palsy. *Neurologist, 9*(6), 311–317.

Mesulam, M. M. (2001). Primary progressive aphasia. *Annals of Neurology, 49*(4), 425–432.

Ogden, R. (2005). Phonetics and social action in agreements and disagreements. *Journal of Pragmatics, 38,* 1752–1775.

Pomerantz, A. (1984). Agreeing and disagreeing with assessments: Some features of preferred/dispreferred turn shapes. In J. Maxwell, J. Atkinson, & J. Heritage (Eds.), *Structures of social action: Studies in conversation analysis* (pp. 57–101). Cambridge, UK: Cambridge University Press.

Raymond, G., & Heritage, J. (2006). The epistemics of social relationships: Owning grandchildren. *Language in Society, 35*(5), 677–705.

Rosen, H. J., Gorno-Tempini, M. L., Goldman, W. P., Perry, R. J., Schuff, N., Weiner, M., ... Miller, B. L. (2002). Patterns of brain atrophy in frontotemporal dementia and semantic dementia. *Neurology, 58*(2), 198–208.

Sacks, H., Schegloff, E., & Jefferson, G. (1974). A simplest systematics for the organization of turn-taking for conversation. *Language, 50*(4), 696–735.

Schegloff, E. (1992). Repair after next turn: The last structurally provided for place for the defense of intersubjectivity in conversation. *American Journal of Sociology, 95,* 1295–1345.

Schegloff, E. (2007). *Sequence organization in interaction: A primer in conversation analysis I* (Vol. 1). Cambridge, UK: Cambridge University Press.
Snowden, J., Neary, D., & Mann, D. (2002). Frontotemporal dementia. *British Journal of Psychiatry, 180,* 140–143.

Recommended Readings

Goodwin, C. (Ed.). (2003). *Conversation and brain damage.* Oxford, UK: Oxford University Press.
Mikesell, L. (2010). Repetitional responses in frontotemporal dementia discourse: Asserting agency or demonstrating confusion? *Discourse Studies, 12*(4), 465–500.
Wray, A. (2010). 'We've had a wonderful, wonderful thing': Formulaic interaction when an expert has dementia. *Dementia, 9*(4), 517–534.

10

Dementia and the Life Course: Examining Cognitive Decline in a Slowly Progressing Degenerative Illness

Michael Halpin and Norann Richard

Learning Objectives

By the end of this chapter, you will be able to:

- Identify how various stages of cognitive decline due to Huntington Disease require adaptations to medical care, including earlier use of objective cognitive testing and active efforts involving family members in medical appointment;
- Better understand dementia as a process that unfolds across the life course, particularly chronic disease-resulting dementia; Researchers, in particular, will learn that different stages of dementia present

M. Halpin (✉)
Department of Sociology and Social Anthropology, Dalhousie University, Halifax, NS, Canada
e-mail: michael.halpin@dal.ca

N. Richard
Clinical Psychologist, CBI Health Centre, Halifax, NS, Canada
e-mail: norichard@cbi.ca

T. Stickle (ed.), *Learning from the Talk of Persons with Dementia*,
The Language of Mental Health, https://doi.org/10.1007/978-3-030-43977-4_10

different challenges for data collection. The authors provide "lessons learned" and best practices for conducting qualitative, in-depth interviews across the life course.
- Gain information on the progression of cognitive decline, especially the numerous ways that cognitive decline might impact communication, and employ different communication strategies and techniques to facilitate better interactions by and with persons with dementia.

This chapter examines dementia across the life course in the context of Huntington Disease (HD), a slowly progressing and degenerative illness. Analysis focuses on five illustrative cases, drawn from a sample of 43 in-depth interviews with members of the HD community. Twenty-four interviews were completed with individuals with the HD mutation and 14 interviews were completed with caregivers. Participants were interviewed across the illness stages of HD, with participants ranging from those that were pre-symptomatic to those requiring managed care. The first author also completed five follow-up interviews (2 dyads, 1 individual interview).

Analysis presents four cross-sections of HD cognitive decline and dementia: (1) the pre-symptomatic period, wherein individuals with the HD-gene express concerns about symptom emergence ($N=5$), (2) early cognitive decline, wherein individuals with HD notice initial symptoms (e.g., difficulties maintaining attention) ($N=6$), (3) advanced symptoms, wherein cognitive impairments cause extreme difficulties in communication ($N=7$), and (4) late-stage symptoms, wherein individuals find communication extremely difficult ($N=5$). Throughout the chapter, the authors reflect on what HD as a case can tell us—clinicians, researchers, caregivers, and patients—about dementia research and care.

Introduction

This chapter reflects on the experiences of individuals living with HD, a genetic, degenerative, and fatal condition. While HD is often characterized by physical symptoms (e.g., chorea), it is also associated with pronounced cognitive symptoms, memory loss, troubles with executive functioning, and difficulties composing speech.

Since the early 1990s, there has been a predictive genetic test for HD (Wexler, 1995). Although the test can determine whether someone has inherited the gene that causes HD, it does not confer diagnosis. Diagnosis is instead based on reaching symptom milestones. However, studies on HD suggest that the cognitive symptoms of HD can appear years prior to official diagnosis (Halpin, 2011). HD symptoms advance until death, which typically occurs 10 to 15 years after formal diagnosis.

Thinking Point

Individuals may experience cognitive symptoms of HD many years prior to a formal diagnosis.

HD is a useful example for reflecting on methodological and health care issues associated with dementia and cognitive decline. First, HD provides a case wherein individuals can discern their future cognitive symptoms via genetic testing. As genetic technologies advance, individuals with other forms of dementia might encounter similar predictive technologies. Second, HD is comparatively slowly progressing, with decades between the time an individual learns of their HD genetic status, when symptoms first appear, and when the individual succumbs to the disease. The long course of HD provides an opportunity for numerous stakeholders (e.g., health care workers, researchers, caregivers, and patients) to reflect on challenges at various stages of the illness.

Our chapter follows HD across the life course. Analysis begins with a case of pre-symptomatic HD, before reviewing cases characteristic of escalating symptom severity. Although we provide an in-depth focus on five cases, data is drawn from a larger interview-based study on HD, consisting of 43 interviews with members of the HD community in British Columbia, Canada. All interviews were conducted by the first author and, consequently, the terms interviewer and first author are used in the text synonymously. We have three aims for each stage of our analysis: (1) to provide a description of relevant cognitive symptoms,

(2) to reflect on challenges or "lessons learned" in conducting qualitative interviews with persons with dementia, and (3) to connect each stage with discrete takeaways for health care professionals who may work with such persons.

"A Different Normal": The Pre-Symptomatic Phase of HD

As noted above, individuals who undergo genetic testing can learn of their HD genetic status decades before symptoms appear. Accordingly, many individuals experience a period when they are gene-positive but symptom-negative, such that they are aware of having the illness-causing gene but have not yet developed symptoms. While these individuals are formally considered "healthy" or pre-symptomatic, they are also aware that on an unknown future date cognitive symptoms will manifest and impact their lives. Our first case reviews such an encounter with HD.

Debbie is a human resources manager and mother of two in her early 40s. Her father and sister have previously been diagnosed with HD, with the former now residing in palliative care. Debbie received her confirmatory genetic test several months prior to her interview, but her neurologist tells her she is currently "symptom free." Accordingly, Debbie maintains her employment, although she struggles to tell her co-workers how she can "have HD" but "not actually have any symptoms." When she does disclose her genetic status, she reports that friends and co-workers are often "devastated" by the news, and they seem to be particularly distressed about "the fact that you lose part of your mental capacities, the executive thinking part." Indeed, the cognitive symptoms are similarly Debbie's biggest concern, as she worries about "keeping [her] mental capacity," asserting that, "it's the mental side that I'm watching really, more than the physical side."

Individuals in Debbie's position (i.e., pre-symptomatic) situate cognitive symptoms as something looming on the horizon, waiting to "take away" their identity, memory, and ability to function. As these individuals do not currently have any symptoms, a disconnect between their genetic status and current physical health can be quite dramatic. Debbie describes how, on some days, she can background her genetic status, whereas on other days, her potential future symptoms emerge to disrupt her life:

> But we're moving along and it's day-to-day and I don't think about [HD]. And then I'll just have a day where something will trigger me and then I don't cope. And it's not like a whole day that I don't cope. I might have an hour or half an hour where I just go "that's it, I don't want to deal with this anymore, I'm tired of dealing with this."

Here, Debbie details how she sometimes cannot "cope" with HD, particularly the feared impact of the aforementioned cognitive symptoms. Nonetheless, HD and its symptoms primarily remain in the background of her life, as she "mov[es] along" and takes things "day-to-day." Indeed, prior to this quote selection, Debbie notes she is considerably more troubled by a recent economic downturn than she is by HD.

In summing up her experience with the pre-symptomatic phase of HD, Debbie emphasizes that her life has, by and large, not yet changed. She is aware that she has a fatal condition that will cause dramatic cognitive decline, but she is equally aware that her day-to-day life is not yet impacted:

> I think I returned to almost normal. I don't think I've ever been normal, I don't think I've ever been quite the same. But I'm not saying that's a bad thing. If anything it's a better thing. Because I tend to look at things a little bit differently. I think it's taught me to examine what I worry about and what I'm concerned about. You learn there's a lot of things that you don't need to be. So almost normal. A different normal.

Debbie argues that, in some ways, HD has improved her life, encouraging her to let go of certain stressors. Her current experience is not reflective of the biographical disruptions that often accompany chronic illness (e.g., Charmaz, 1991), nor is she in "denial" about her disease or its consequences. Instead, Debbie is navigating a period of pre-patienthood (Timmermans & Buchbinder, 2010), a space between health and illness that she sees as "normal" but "a different normal." Accordingly, in terms of social scientific methodology, the interview with Debbie is not remarkable in relation to her cognitive experience or status. Indeed, we suggest the methodological takeaway, particularly in terms of recruitment and sampling strategy, is that an individual's health status might or might not be salient to them regardless of what researchers might presume about someone's response to predictive testing.

For health care providers, Debbie's experience can serve as a reminder to investigate patient's perceptions of their symptoms. While Debbie herself did not report becoming overly fixated on the possibility of future impairments, this remained a source of concern for her. Depending on individuals' self-perceptions and the extent to which their identity is focused on their intellectual or cognitive abilities, anxiety over future decline might take on a more significant role in their lives. Indeed, this worry can in turn lead to increased hypervigilance to the perceived early signs of cognitive decline, and may result in normal lapses in memory and concentration being interpreted in a particularly negative fashion. Medical providers may want to provide reassurance and reminders about typical fluctuations in cognitive abilities.

"I'm Not Disabled, I'm Under-Employed": Emergence of Initial HD Symptoms

The second case we review is based on an interview completed with Scott, a Canadian/English citizen in his late 40s. Scott spent the last several years of his life working overseas, earning a considerable wage. He returned to Canada after discovering his sister had been diagnosed with HD. Upon his arrival, he also received a confirmatory genetic test. Moreover, Scott's subsequent neurological assessment revealed that he was already manifesting symptoms, and he was conferred a formal HD diagnosis. Scott was unable to return home, leaving behind his romantic partner and his job. The interview with Scott occurs several months after his diagnosis.

Scott and the first author (i.e., interviewer) had numerous informal and often philosophical conversations about genetic science, HD, and death, prior to their interview. From the interviewer's perspective, Scott, like Debbie, had no discernable HD symptoms. Based on Scott's self-assessment, his interactions with the interviewer, as well as indications from health care workers, the first author suspected his HD symptoms would not impact their interview. As the following material demonstrates, this was not the case.

The first author visits Scott in his downtown apartment, where he lives alone. The apartment is small and well-kept, decorated with paintings and sculptures. Scott is an avid computer-gamer and his personal computer occupies a prominent position in the living room. At the beginning of the interview, Scott notes he is keeping an active social life, running "three times a week, rain or shine." Furthermore, to ward off HD symptoms, Scott says "I challenge my mind" by "teaching myself new things… I practice math, languages. Just as a form of interest. I teach myself new skills." However, Scott also notes he has been "feeling depressed" lately, telling the interviewer, "I woke up angry this morning." When asked if his depression is related to HD, Scott responds, "No, depression has been with me for a while."

As the interview begins, Scott discloses, "My brain says this can't really be happening to me." When asked to elaborate, Scott says, "I was just on the ocean… with my amore." The next thing he knows he is "back in Canada" and "under employed." Reflecting on these large life changes, Scott says, "When I meet with the psychiatrist, I can rationalize it, and see it for what it is. But when I leave his office, I think: I don't want to walk down this road." Scott has applied for jobs in Canada but has not received any return calls; consequently, his daughter and health care workers tell him he needs to sign up for disability benefits to protect his finances. Raising a common refrain in the interview, Scott argues, "I'm not disabled! I'm under employed (laughs)." Scott further suggests that an economic downturn in his industry, rather than HD symptoms, is keeping him out of work. Summing up the tensions between himself, his daughter, and health care workers, Scott notes, "I have one foot in one world, one foot in another world."

From a data collection perspective, all is proceeding very well, as Scott thoughtfully reflects on open-ended questions, providing vivid details on the dilemmas he faces. However, the first author is also noticing that Scott's voice has begun to slur, a symptom that has not appeared in any of their previous interactions.

The first tangible breakdown in the interview occurs approximately at the twenty-minute mark. Scott is discussing how his wife, who passed away from cancer, modeled how someone could live with a fatal prognosis, stating "she was very good at demonstrating being diagnosed with something and accepting it with the fullness of your being," while adding, "but [HD] is very different." The first author asks Scott to elaborate. After a brief pause, Scott responds, "Being left-handed has been no treat, you know. Everyone thinks you're incompetent."

As this response seems tangential and unconnected to the question, the interviewer is slightly confused about how to advance, and interprets Scott's response as humorous. They both begin to laugh. The interviewer then attempts to reframe the question, asking Scott what his experience with his wife taught him "about dealing with serious illness." Scott takes up the topic stating, "I learned we are all infinite," adding that her physical decline inspired him to take up running, now a major part of his life. Scott and the first author compare cancer and HD for the next several minutes, with Scott summing up his perspective by stating, "Acceptance isn't accepting death. It's accepting the disease. And what the disease can do to you." With the interview seemingly back on track, the first author situates the breakdown as a typical miscommunication, which often occurs during in-depth interviews, particularly when sensitive topics are addressed.

Additional breakdowns occur as the interview progresses. For instance, a central component of the interview guide is a "grand tour" question (Spradley, 1979): a common qualitative technique that asks participants to walk the interviewer through an aspect of their experience, in this case, the day Scott learned he had HD. There are numerous breakdowns during Scott's response to this question. First, Scott discusses meeting a psychiatrist prior to learning of his genetic status.

While describing the meeting, Scott begins a tangent about his life overseas that lasts several minutes. When Scott completes the tangent, the first author uses a probing question (Weiss, 1995) about the psychiatrist to return to where they "left off." Scott recalls the psychiatrist's concerns that he might commit suicide if he received a confirmatory result. Scott assures the psychiatrist that, as a survivor of suicide, he would never take his own life. The psychiatrist then opens an envelope containing Scott's testing results, and discloses that Scott, indeed, has HD. Here, Scott again leaves the topic of the grand tour question and returns to discussing his time overseas. Indeed, the interview, much like Scott's assessment of his life at the moment, has "one foot in one world, one foot in another world."

At this point, the first author notes Scott has no difficulty discussing topics, even very sensitive topics, but is encountering challenges with remaining on a topic. Adapting his questioning, the interviewer begins to take judicious notes on Scott's responses, which he uses as "anchors" to return to Scott's responses after each diversion. The interviewer drops the formality of the "grand tour" questions, moving to a more conversational approach that is tailored to oscillations between talk on international travel, HD, death, employment, and symptoms.

While Scott's cognitive symptoms were not apparent in any previous conversation with the first author, or at the beginning of their interview, they emerged over the duration of a more structured conversation. Indeed, the interviewer finally becomes aware of the extent of his initial ignorance of Scott's cognitive symptoms only after Scott tells a joke partway through their interview. Picking up his glasses, Scott says "I lost this arm from my glasses. And I found it, over there on the carpet. But the thing is, I lost it at the [HD] clinic! What's it doing over there! (laughs)." The interviewer replies, "Change of address, huh?" Scott shakes his head, "No, it's just a reminder that we're here for a short period of time and then we move on." For Scott, his memory lapse with the glasses is indicative of his advancing HD symptoms. For the first author, Scott's lapse reveals his struggles with memory loss, which had not been evident prior to the interview.

From a qualitative methodological perspective, Scott's experience emphasizes issues with context and dementia symptoms. During informal or brief conversations, it would be difficult to discern Scott's cognitive symptoms. However, over the course of a two-hour interview that covers personal topics, experiences, and reflections, the cognitive symptoms become more salient. The formal interview challenged the first author's assumptions of minimal cognitive symptoms based on prior conversation. Thus, this provides a lesson for interviewers to consider that cognitive impairments might vary depending on context and that varying types of interactional tasks may bring different levels of impairment into relief. Additionally, to adjust to the situation, the interviewer extensively jotted touchstone or "anchor" statements that he could use to return to the prior topic of the interview.

Research Tips

1. Be aware that the extent of cognitive impairments may vary according to context and situation and be prepared to deviate between structured interview protocols and informal conversational exchanges
2. Take detailed notes to help return to earlier topics when participants may have difficulties remaining focused.

With regard to health care providers, Scott's case serves as an important reminder to employ objective measures of cognitive ability. Professionals can often rely on their initial patient impressions, especially given the often-limited time available for medical appointments. Professionals might not recognize impairment like Scott's, as such impairment can be masked by education, extensive vocabulary, or good social skills. Accordingly, standardized employment of brief empirically supported cognitive screening tests, such as the St. Louis University Mental Status Examination (SLUMS; Feliciano et al., 2013), across all patients with particular risk factors might be a helpful way to better detect the early signs of impairment among individuals who might initially appear cognitively fit. These measures can be used in combination with the more subjective aspects of evaluation, including open-ended questions, queries about the patients' perceptions of their symptoms, and follow-up questions about the results of objective testing. This approach can help clinicians obtain a more comprehensive picture of an individual's symptomology than an exclusive focus on objective testing or patient's self-reports.

Thinking Point

Objective cognitive screening can be beneficial to add for patients whose cognitive impairments may not be immediately apparent in short medical appointments.

"He Needs a Long Time to Digest": Pronounced Symptoms in HD

Our third case is based on an interview completed with Markus, a Dutch immigrant and a retired construction-site manager in his mid-60s. Markus had received his HD diagnosis 10 years prior to the interview and had received a confirmatory genetic test 8 years prior to that diagnosis.

The first author visits both Markus and his wife Agatha for a joint interview at their rural home. After the interviewer stated he had no preference of participant order, the couple decided that Markus should be interviewed first, with Agatha retiring to another room. Before the interview, Markus made some tea in his large, brightly lit kitchen while fending off the attention of his two large Labrador retrievers. During this conversation, the first author noted Markus slurred his speech and had chorea in his limbs, particularly his legs. That said, Markus and the first author had a long and lively conversation about Canadian politics, with Markus providing a detailed and passionate assessment of a minority party's rare parliamentary maneuver that had the potential to reshape political power. Based on Markus' political acumen, the interviewer anticipated a spirited interaction.

The interview begins with several close-ended questions asking the participant to recall specific dates. Markus advanced through these questions readily. However, the interview encountered difficulties during the "grand tour" question (detailed above). After the interviewer poses the question, Markus responds, "do I remember what day it was? No,

I don't." When the first author clarifies by asking Markus to "tell me about the day you found out you had HD, in as much detail as you can recall," Markus replies, "it was in the old children's hospital, I had to walk the long hallway to get to the office (long pause). The doctor had an envelope and he opened it. [He said] my uncle had that gene and I had it also." Once completing this statement, Markus stopped speaking and the first author assumed he was anticipating the next question.

After the long, flowing conversation on politics, the first author was confused by the comparatively abrupt answers. Pausing to reframe his approach, he attempts to "walk" Markus through the question using probing questions. The first author begins by asking Markus about his reaction to the doctor's pronouncement. Markus responds, "My reaction? I told him that I was (pause) relieved. I was smiling actually. In a way I was relieved that I knew what was going to happen." Noting that Markus was "relieved" about a diagnosis that many might find distressing, the interviewer asks him to elaborate. Markus then tells a long story about being impacted by mysterious symptoms that no physician could explain. Despite the initial difficulties, the interview seems back on course.

The challenges with the interview return when the first author completes the grand tour question and raises a new topic. Here, Markus' responses again seem brief, abrupt, and potentially incomplete. For example, the first author asks, "So did you know Huntington's was in your family before the genetic test?" Markus responds, "Uh yeah, but. I can't. Not. I got con-con-confronted with it in 1987." This is the first time the date 1987 appears in the interview, so the first author asks, "What happened in 1987?" Markus replies:

> An uncle of mine. He had all kinds of. He said. And symptoms. The doctor did not know what was going on with him. He spent time in several hospitals. Until they finally found out what he had. But no one else in the family had it. And then, looking back, he must have gotten it from my grandfather. And my grandfather passed away in his early 50s. So even if he had it. He passed away from a stomach condition.

At this stage, the first author is having difficulty parsing Markus' responses, which is considerably more challenging during real-time conversation without the aid of a transcript. It now sounds like Markus has an uncle who was diagnosed with HD before he received his own genetic test, yet that would appear to complicate Markus' story of the challenges he encountered pursuing a diagnosis. As such, the interviewer is unsure if Markus' uncle was diagnosed first or if Markus is instead suggesting that his uncle must have had HD, based on his symptoms and Markus' genetic status.

In an attempt to clarify Markus' responses, the interviewer asks a different style of question, elaborating his question by providing Markus with several potential response options: "So between 1987 and your gene test in 1992, given your family history, did you think you had the mutation, did you think you didn't have it?" The question works with the premise that Markus knew about his uncle's genetic status, and asks him to reflect on his genetic risk prior to his own predictive testing. Markus responds:

> First, um like, for like (pause) to early (pause) very late 80s, we knew it was there, but we didn't, we knew that I was here, and of course, my uncle, he uh, he was diagnosed at the time. But uh yeah. But he did with work. He didn't look that bad. The only thing he had was trouble with his balance.

The answer is difficult to interpret. Although the first author adapted his approach several times, he is encountering more difficulties with the interview, as Markus' answers are harder to decipher as the interview advances.

As it turns out, part of the difficulty is that the author is working with an incorrect premise that Markus has difficulty correcting: that he knew of his uncle's HD prior to his own genetic test. Instead, based on a correction Markus makes later in the interview, what he is aiming to reveal is that his uncle became ill in 1987 and, in retrospect, this was the emergence of HD. By and large, the interview is characterized by these types of communication difficulties until its conclusion.

The interviewer then directs his questions to Agatha, Markus' spouse. Following standard ethics board protocol, the first author is prohibited from discussing Markus' interview with his wife. However, inadvertently, Agatha's interview provides numerous insights into the communication difficulties the first author encountered. For example, he asks Agatha what symptoms she has noticed in Markus:

> His comprehension is different. Maybe he'll understand but it may take him twelve or twenty-four hours sometimes before I get an answer back. Like to explain him something like, "these are the options," then he needs a long time to digest, process that. The best way to approach it is to just give him one scenario at the time, like you know, never offer him, "would you like a glass of wine or a glass of beer?" Just say, "you want a glass of wine?" I get a "no," "you want a glass of beer?" I get a "yes" right?

Returning to the interview with Markus (above), the interviewer provides Markus with questions with multiple response options, "Did you think you had the mutation, did you think you didn't have it?" Based on Agatha's insights, the interviewer has constructed exactly the type of question that might be difficult for Markus.

Agatha similarly sheds light on Markus' seemingly abrupt answers, stating, "He struggles with the fact that he can't fully express what he thinks. So some things might come out the wrong way in a brief sentence, whereas he can't totally bring across his total way of feeling." Rather than providing an abrupt or disinterested response to the first author's questions, Agatha's interview suggests Markus might have been frustrated by feeling like he incompletely expressed his opinion. While the first author took Markus' silence as a sign to move onto another topic, the silence could have been interpreted more aptly as a lengthy pause and opportunity for Markus to collect his thoughts, elaborate his point, and provide a more complete response.

Part of the difficulty the first author encountered was the contrast between Markus' discussion of politics and their formal interview. At least initially, the author assumed Markus was disinterested in the interview due to the comparatively brief responses. However, Agatha once again inadvertently clarifies the situation, situating politics as somewhat of a "special case" for Markus:

> He gets very, very alert very aggressive when it's about politics. Oh man, yeah, we'll go somewhere and I begged him last week, "please don't talk about politics," he gets so aggressive about it. And, he'll really know his stuff, that's the thing.

In Agatha's view, while Markus might have difficulty formulating responses and choosing among options, this is not the case with politics where he "really knows his stuff." Indeed, rather than facilitating his communication, Agatha sometimes feels like she has to discourage Markus from discussing the topic.

In terms of qualitative methods, Markus' interview, as with Scott's, stresses the importance of not extrapolating a participant's cognitive symptoms across different domains of conversation. Viewing Markus and Agatha's interviews together also suggest that the interpersonal cues that qualitative interviewers often rely on, such as interpreting lengthy pauses as the completion of a response, do not necessarily capture the experience of dementia symptoms. Similarly, clarifying questions by providing a range of potential response options might complicate, rather than simplify, the question, as asking a participant to select among different response options might require increased cognitive effort.

For health professionals, Markus' interview highlights the importance of involving family members in care whenever possible. To balance issues of consent and cognitive decline, professionals should seek a patient's consent to involve a family member in ongoing care at the time of any initial diagnosis that might involve future cognitive impairment. Furthermore, patient's family members might be able to offer insights on symptomology that the patient is not able to self-report. Given debates surrounding the accuracy of symptom measurements during the advanced stages of cognitive illness (e.g., assessment of depression severity in individuals with advanced HD, see Paulsen et al., 2005), they can also help the provider become aware when self-reports are not providing an accurate picture of daily functioning. In addition, this example also highlights the need for providers to use a variety of question styles when interacting with individuals with cognitive impairments. For some, such as Markus, simple close-ended questions may be easier for the patient to comprehend and may allow a more effective use of time. However, for others, open-ended questions may provide helpful follow-up or a chance to elaborate on concerns that may be otherwise forgotten or neglected.

"I Shouldn't Be Here": Advanced HD Symptoms

The last cases are drawn from interviews the first author completed with individuals with advanced HD. While this section returns to Markus and Agatha, the first example is an interview with Jim, who was residing in a care facility at the time of the interview. Although the author was concerned about Jim's ability to participate, his wife informed the first author that Jim was high functioning and very excited about research. She also stated the decision to move Jim to a care facility was more influenced by her difficulty in providing adequate in-home support than Jim's symptoms.

The first author met Jim, a retired naval pilot in his early 70s, at his private care facility. The first author explains who he is when he first arrives, and Jim replies that he "knows all about [the interview]." Jim has notable chorea in his hands, as well as trouble moving and the first author helps him transition to his wheelchair for the interview. As the first author turns on his recorders, Jim states, "I don't have Huntington's Disease." Concerned that this statement might indicate severe cognitive difficulties, the interviewer asks, "Can you elaborate on that for me?" Jim reframes, "Oh, I have it. But it's a very minor case." Given that Jim is in his early 70s and the majority of individuals with HD succumb to symptoms in their 40s–50s, Jim's assessment seems plausible to the first author. Nonetheless, the first author asks for clarification, and Jim compares himself to another resident with HD, who is "constantly screaming and thrashing about." Content with the answer, the first author begins with the interview.

The interview begins uneventfully. The first author asks Jim several close-ended demographic questions that Jim easily answers. The interviewer then asks Jim the "grand tour" question, which asks Jim to reflect on the day he discovered he had HD:

> The doctor suspected that there was something weird going on, not - so he lined up a - a - he figured it'd be Huntington's because he couldn't figure out a symptom for the kind of things that I had. So I went to [university] and I got checked into [the clinic], and ah, that was about 3 to 4 years ago, ah 4 years. So then they did a test, and ah... h'm, yeah they did a test and ah, at the very worst they figured it was a minor ah... mm... how did they describe it? "Minor HD." Ah... so I took the whole family and I sat them down and said "some idiots have figured out that I have Huntington's" and, so it was not well received 'cause they know me, they know me and they didn't see that bullshit.

Jim provides an apt answer to the "grand tour" question, although he also seems skeptical about his diagnostic status. Given that Jim is residing in managed care and has notable chorea, the author plans to unpack Jim's diagnostic skepticism in follow-up questions.

When the first author begins to ask Jim about his perspective on his diagnosis, his responses become exceedingly brief. One difficulty is that, in attempt to invite elaboration, the interviewer replaces his open-ended questions with close-ended questions. For example, the following exchange starts with an open-ended question ("what were your thoughts...") but then switches to close-ended:

```
MH:    So what were your thoughts on being told that you were
       sick when you weren't sick?
Jim:   Well I had ah every specialist in town (inaudible),
       um... mm...
MH:    Did they give you a genetic test for it?
Jim:   Mm. Yeah.
MH:    Okay.
Jim:   Yeah, they did.
MH:    And did that say that you had it?
Jim:   Yeah.
MH:    Okay.
Jim:   But I was - it was such a low-level thing -
MH:    Do you remember the number they gave you?
Jim:   Hm.
MH:    The number of CAG repeats, I think it is?
Jim:   ah - and the number is six, would that make sense?
MH:    Okay. Okay ... how do you think being told you have HD
        has changed your life? has changed your life?
Jim:   Nothing.
MH:    Nothing?
Jim:   Nothing.
```

The open-ended question that starts this exchange addresses a central paradox of the HD experience, namely that someone can have the gene for HD but not yet manifest any of the symptoms (see Halpin, 2018). The question picks up on Jim's perspective that he was not ill at the time of his diagnosis. Jim's response is somewhat tangential, focusing on the number of specialists he saw, potentially in an effort to secure a diagnosis to explain his symptoms. Suspecting that the specialists might be geneticists, and attempting to prompt a longer response, the first author provides Jim with a close-ended probing question, "did they give you a genetic test for [HD]?" While such close-ended probes can elicit elaborated responses, Jim responds to the close-ended question as it is framed, providing a simple "yes" to the interviewer's "yes or no" question. Attempting to produce additional details on his testing experience, the interviewer asks Jim if he recalls his CAG repeat count. While individuals with symptomatic HD have a minimum of 36 repeats, Jim tentatively suggests his count is "six." Caught off guard by this response, the interviewer attempts to change the topic by asking a broad and open-ended question, which produces another single-word answer.

The remainder of the interview unfolds similar to this selection, wherein Jim provides a brief or tangential response to an open-ended question but is able to detail his account through extensive close-ended follow-ups. However, Jim also begins to have more pronounced memory troubles, asserting several times that he is 65, rather than in his 70s, and has just recently retired as a pilot. While the first author did cobble together a basic sense of Jim's narrative or experience through the responses to these numerous close-ended questions, the responses largely lack the detail needed for analyses.

The first author's interview with Jim highlights several methodological challenges for qualitative interviewers. First, individuals with advanced HD encounter difficulty answering in-depth and open-ended questions. While this wasn't the case for the first open-ended question Jim was asked, it became an issue in the remainder of the interview. Second, an individual's family members (e.g., Jim's wife) are not necessarily aware of how cognitive symptoms might impact an individual's ability to respond to an open-ended question, but they may offer insights. An issue here is that qualitative interviews are often described as "conversational" to alleviate participants' apprehensions and to emphasize the semi-structured nature of the interview. However, describing an interview as "conversational" or "like a conversation" in the context of interviewing person with dementia obscures the often demanding nature of open-ended questions.

Given these difficulties, it might appear reasonable to avoid interviews with individuals with marked cognitive symptoms of HD. However, Jim and individuals with comparable symptom presentations were explicitly interested in participating in the first author's research. The tension between participant interest and interview quality raises issues of inclusion and concerns about ruling an individual out of the research process based on assumptions of neurotypicality. That said, interviews that are not likely to produce data suitable for analysis also carry costs for researchers.

To resolve this tension, and to balance inclusivity, data quality, and bioethics, we suggest conducting tandem interviews when participants have pronounced cognitive symptoms. In this scenario, a family member or trusted acquaintance provides context-sensitive interactional expertise vis-à-vis communicating with a person with dementia. The first author completed two such interviews, one of which was a follow-up interview with Agatha and Markus nearly a decade after the initial interview. We use this encounter to detail the utility of tandem interviews.

Before the interview begins, the first author tells Markus and Agatha that he will "let [them] take the lead" in deciding how to respond to a question but that he will make sure both partners have opportunities to speak to each interview item. The first author begins by asking the duo, "How have things changed from the first interview?" Markus takes the lead in responding:

```
MH:  All I can say is that I'm glad because my son got tested
     last year.
A:   On no, that was a long time ago.
MH:  Was it three years ago?
A:   I thought he got tested before they got married?
MH:  Oh, ok, that's right. And his test was negative.
A:   And then they had a little baby girl, so both of our
     children are negative, in the positive sense.
```

Markus orients the duo's answer to the question by highlighting the most notable development for himself: neither of his children inherited the gene for HD, which means none of his children or grandchildren will develop the condition. Agatha intercedes to correct Markus' error in recalling the specific time his last son received his testing and, after the correction, joins Markus in emphasizing the "positive" news that their children do not have the HD gene. The remainder of the interview unfolds in a similar pattern, with Markus providing an initial response, while Agatha fills in the details. When Agatha speaks, Markus similarly remains engaged, nodding and murmuring "yes, yes" as she recounts events and experiences. Although Markus is considerably impacted by the symptoms of HD, the three of us have a nearly two-hour interview. Indeed, unlike the first author's interview with Jim, or his first interview with Markus, he is able to document the vivid and detailed accounts needed for qualitative analyses.

> **Research Tip**
>
> Tandem interviews with persons with dementia and their family may help to obtain the most detailed and accurate responses to questions.

For health care professionals, these examples again highlight the importance of involving family members in medical appointments whenever possible. Information gathering and symptom documenting can be especially challenging with individuals who struggle with memory and attention to detail, and as such, loved ones can often provide the context cues that are vital to medical providers to allow for accurate diagnosis and treatment. However, it is also vital to emphasize the dignity of the individuals with cognitive impairments. As done in the interview with Markus and Agatha, it is important to allow the patient themselves a chance to answer and express concerns, as despite difficulties with expression, they remain the expert on their own personal experiences. It is unfortunately common for persons with dementia to be treated in a paternalistic fashion or for providers to direct questions at family members, rather than the patient directly; it is crucial in patient-centered care for the patient to remain the focal point in the medical appointment.

Summary

Huntington Disease provides both an opportunity to view dementia as a process and a means to reflect on how different stages of dementia confront researchers and health care providers with varying challenges. With the first case, Debbie, dementia is a specter, such that the prospective impact of the disease can be haunting, but its effects are still abstract and ephemeral. At this stage, it is paramount for interviewers to follow the participants' definitions in order to understand how they might see themselves as "different" but also "normal." The second case, Scott, emphasizes the fluidity of dementia symptoms, which might or might not be salient at all phases of the interview, and underscores the need for researchers to plan or adapt to variability in cognitive issues as the interview unfolds. A takeaway from the third case, Markus, is that researchers should be cautious about generalizing between types of talk (e.g., formal and informal) and draw on the conversational "tricks of the trade" used by spouses and family members of persons with dementia to improve an interview. The last cases—Jim and subsequent tandem interview with Markus and Agatha—outline difficulties and strategies for interviewing individuals with advanced dementia. At this stage, we suggest tandem interviews to expand participation while also attending to data quality.

These in-depth interviews also provide a unique viewpoint on the variable nature of cognitive decline in HD, which can be informative for medical providers who encounter this process. For instance, in reflecting on the experience of Debbie, who feared future cognitive decline despite showing no present evidence of such symptoms, medical providers may become more conscientious of the role that a feared future plays in patient's present-day concerns. Remaining sensitive to these concerns and the impact they may have on patient's own attention to their cognitive performance is useful not only in the case of HD, but also for patients who may have a strong history of dementia in their family, or who have neurological conditions that might or might not cause cognitive issues (e.g., multiple sclerosis). Additionally, the case of Jim, along with the repeat interviews with Agatha and Markus, it is important to emphasize the benefits of family engagement as a central part of healthcare for individuals with a variety of cognitive impairments; indeed, the benefits of such an approach suggest that planning for the family to take an active role could be started sooner in the degenerative process.

Practical Highlights

1. Take copious notes while interviewing persons with dementia to ensure topics are not obscured by tangents or diversions.
2. Use family members' and loved one's experience and expertise communicating with persons with dementia to inform your strategy for an in-depth interview.
3. Consider conducting tandem interviews with a family member/loved one and the person with dementia with advanced symptoms to balance research inclusivity with data quality.
4. As cognitive symptoms may not always be evident within a short medical visit, objective cognitive testing can be helpful to better detect symptoms for HD gene positive patients or anyone at risk for future cognitive decline.
5. While persons with dementia should always be treated as the experts on their symptoms, health care professionals should plan more proactively for the future involvement of family members in medical appointments for patients at risk of cognitive decline.

References

Charmaz, K. (1991). *Good days, bad days: The self in chronic illness and time.* New Brunswick, NJ: Rutgers University Press.

Feliciano, L., Horning, S. M., Kiebe, K. J., Anderson, S. L., Cornwell, R. E., & Davos, H. P. (2013). Utility of the SLUMS as a cognitive screening tool among a nonveteran sample of older adults. *American Journal of Geriatric Psychiatry, 21*(7), 623–630.

Halpin, M. (2011). Diagnosis, psychiatry, and neurology: The case of Huntington disease. *Social Science and Medicine, 73*(6), 858–865.

Halpin, M. (2018). Science and suffering: Genetics and the lived experience of illness. *Social Problem, 65*(3), 360–376.

Paulsen, J. S., Nehl, C., Hoth, K. F., Kanz, J. E., Benjamin, M., Conybeare, R., ... Turner, B. (2005). Depression and stages of Huntington's disease. *The Journal of Neuropsychiatry and Clinical Neurosciences, 17*(4), 496–502.

Spradley, J. P. (1979). *The ethnographic interview.* Belmont, CA: Waveland Press.

Timmermans, S., & Buchbinder, M. (2010). Patients-in-waiting: Living between sickness and health in the genomics era. *Journal of Health and Social Behavior, 51*(4), 408–423.

Weiss, R. S. (1995). *Learning from strangers: The art and method of qualitative interview studies*. New York, NY: The Free Press.

Wexler, A. (1995). *Mapping fate: A memoir of family, risk, and genetic research*. New York, NY: Times Books.

Recommended Readings

Johnson, A. R., & Paulsen, J. S. (2014). *Understanding behavior in Huntington's disease: A guide for professionals*. New York, NY: The Huntington Disease Society of America.

Tarapata, K., & Murrary, C. (2011). *A caregiver's guide to Huntington's disease*. New York, NY: The Huntington Disease Society of America.

11

Public and Private Spaces in Residential Care for Older People

Gunilla Jansson

Learning Objectives

By the end of this chapter, you will be able to:

- Identify the challenges associated with the ambiguity of the private and public spaces in residential care facilities;
- Recognize methods by which care workers and others can manage these challenges.

G. Jansson (✉)
Department of Swedish Language and Multilingualism, Stockholm University, Stockholm, Sweden
e-mail: Gunilla.Jansson@su.se

T. Stickle (ed.), *Learning from the Talk of Persons with Dementia*,
The Language of Mental Health, https://doi.org/10.1007/978-3-030-43977-4_11

Introduction

Disability can necessitate care that involves transgressing customary social rules concerning privacy. In particular, when disability calls for a move to a residential facility, the individual's private territory becomes the workplace of another. While the home bathroom is one place where private matters such as bathing, washing, and bodily excreting are accomplished and in a person's ordinary home are commonly done alone; and, while one's living room is a public place within a home, it still has symbols, like decorations, that indicate privacy in terms of residents' right to control this space. In a residential care center, boundaries between private and public—of both the bathroom and living room—become unclear.

In this chapter, I present observations on care workers' and residents' negotiating public and private spheres in residential care facilities for older people in Sweden. I focus on the private bathroom and the common living room to shed light on the complexity and diversity of the residential care facility as a semi-public environment, a place both for institutional care and personal life. The ambiguity of these two spaces and the associated challenges has been emphasized in the research literature on care work (Hauge & Heggen, 2008; Twigg, 1999, 2000). Using conversation analysis (Sidnell & Stivers, 2013) and ethnographic observations (Hammersley & Atkinson, 2007), I investigate how care staff and residents more or less successfully manage the dual nature of the residential care facility as private and public space (Fig. 11.1).

Extract 1 illustrates the ambiguity to which this chapter is devoted. It is taken from a conversation between a resident (R) Siri and a care worker (CW) Anna during a morning care session at a dementia unit in a Swedish residential care facility. The care activity takes place in the resident's private bathroom. Siri has been toileting and is at present standing at the basin washing her hands. Anna is assisting the resident with small tasks. In line 1, Anna takes a towel and hands it to Siri.

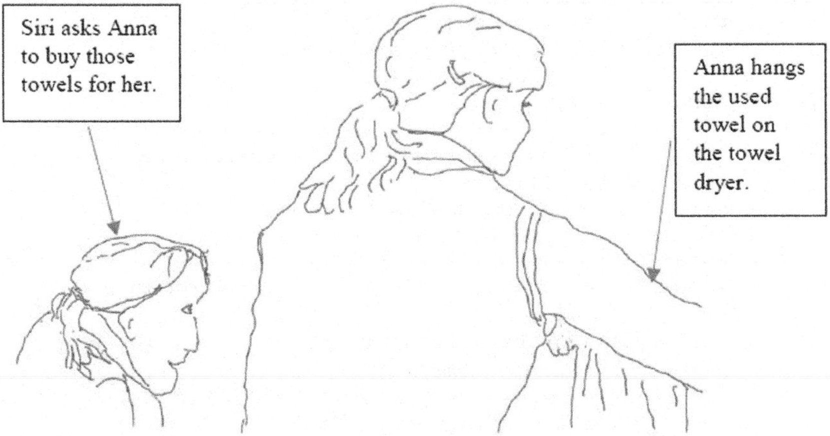

Fig. 11.1 Anna hangs towel (*Source* Author)

Extract 1: Ambiguity in the residential care environment

01.	Anna:	varsågod
	(CW)	*here you are*
		+hands over a towel to Siri+
02.	Siri:	tack
	(R)	*thank you*
03.		(2.0)
04.	Siri:	va söta dom här handdukarna e
		how pretty these towels are
05.	Anna:	javisst e'rom gulliga
		yes they are cute aren't they
06.	Siri:	såna här skulle ja behö- (.) kan du köpa nåra
		I could use some of the- (.) could you buy some
07.		såna här till min bo- (.) privata bostad
		I need that at my ho- (.) private home
08.	Anna:	ja de kan vi göra
		yes we can do that
09.	Siri:	dom var jättesöta tycker ja
		they are super pretty I think
		**holds the towel in her hands------->*
10.	Anna:	m:m (0.5) jättefin färg e're
		m:m (0.5) a super nice color
	siri:	--------------------------------->

11.	Siri:	(xxx) ja dom e söta
		(xxx) *yes they are pretty*
		---------------------------*
12.	Anna:	ja↑:
		yes
13.		*+hangs the towel on the towel dryer--->*
		#fig.11.1
14.	Siri:	de kan du skaffa till mej
		you can buy those for me
	Anna:	----------------------------->
15.	Anna:	de kan ja skaffa till dej (.) om inte du vill följa
		I can buy them for you (.) *if you don't want to come*
		------------------------------+
		me å handla
		with me and go shopping

This extract exemplifies care staff and residents managing the ambiguous boundaries between public and private spheres in a care facility. Siri in Extract 1, who is diagnosed with dementia, needs help with her daily hygiene in her private bathroom space that is simultaneously Anna's workspace. While asking for and receiving help, Siri and Anna talk about towels (line 04). Talking about something other than the body, such as a physical object in the surrounding environment, in the current case a towel, takes away the focus from the care activity (Ridell, 2008) and the breach between private and public space.

What is noteworthy is not only the use of language as distraction, but also the way the resident refers to her presently living at the care facility as temporary, with the towels as alien objects that do not belong to her. The towels have been purchased by the care staff and paid for with the resident's money. As such, they are meant to be seen as the resident's belongings. In the sequence above, Anna and Siri praise the towels, but the towels are portrayed as no one's private possession. The fact that Siri asks the care worker to buy this specific kind of towel for her private home (lines 06–07) supports the notion that home is someplace else, and that her place at the residential care facility is not home. In line 14, Siri asks Anna to buy those towels for her 'real' home: 'de kan du skaffa till mej' (*you can buy those for me*). Anna's reply, 'de kan jag skaffa till dej' (*I can buy them for you*) contributes to the portrayal of the towels as semi-public objects, detached from personal ownership, and something one can observe and admire from a distance, something Siri admires and would like to have as her own.

Viewing one's place at the residential care facility as only temporary is a common strategy used among residents to create a sense of control and belonging (Falk, Wijk, & Falk, 2012). Despite the fact that Siri has lived at the care facility for several years, and will probably do so for the rest of her life, her old residence would always be her home. Even though Anna did her best to personalize Siri's room (e.g., towels), Siri's sense of 'home' lies outside the institution.

Over the last decades, the negative effects of institutionalized care have become better understood; from this, the recognition of older people's need for and right to privacy has developed. As a consequence, attempts have been made to profile residential care facilities as real homes. One measure has been to arrange common living rooms with elements that can be seen as typical symbols that mark a living room in a home. Another has been to design small-scale environments with single rooms and private bathrooms that make room for residents' personal belongings. Despite these attempts, research indicates that problems associated with the institutionalization of older people's care, such as loss of privacy, remain (Heinemann, 2011; Jansson, 2016), and residents are limited in maintaining privacy or exerting control (Hauge & Heggen, 2008)—all of which are key characteristics of a home according to social anthropologists (e.g., Douglas, 1991). The effects of such loss can be the cause of both physical and mental decline (Williams, 2011). In line with this argumentation, Falk et al. (2012, p. 1006) advocate for a clearer demarcation between the public and private, which would provide less ambiguous signals to care staff and residents.

In prior ethnographic research, residential care has often been described as negative (Allan & Crow, 1989; Goffman, 1961; Grainger, 1993; I. Higgins, 1998; J. Higgins, 1989; Lee-Treweek, 1994, 1998; Makoni & Grainger, 2002; Nussbaum, 1993; Twigg, 2000). In Goffman's (1961) terms, the residential home is a 'total institution', a stigmatized world where the person is made subject to collective regimes. The literature on residential care accounts for a world where private space such as bathrooms 'become some of the most public rooms where personal territory and dignity are frequently invaded' (J. Higgins, 1989, p. 145), and where residents 'have few personal possessions with which to maintain their sense of self' (Twigg, 2000, p. 134). It is particularly the absence of privacy, the power to shut the door and exclude the public world outside, that is described as one of the most disliked aspects of living in residential homes (Allan & Crow, 1989). In contrast to previously reported negative aspects of life in residential homes, this chapter highlights the brighter side of institutional care. The purpose of the chapter is to account for methods that care workers adopt to order space in a way that maintains a sense of privacy and dignity for the resident.

After discussing the data, the analysis is divided into two sections. In section "The Ambiguous Space of the Bathroom" (Extracts 2–5), I demonstrate how care workers negotiate their presence in the resident's private bathroom during morning care, and how they manage the body as spatially arranged according to gradations of privacy (cf. Twigg, 1999). The setting in section "The Ambiguous Space of the Common Living Room" (Extracts 6–7) is the common living room. I describe the strategies by which a resident creates a sense of home and privacy in the common living room and demonstrate how this leads to problematic situations that the care staff has to manage. Finally, I give a short summary of the practical highlights of the study.

Data

Data are drawn from two larger projects on communicative practices in older people's care in Sweden headed by the author of this chapter (Jansson & Nikolaidou, 2013; Jansson, Wadensjö, & Plejert, 2017). Ethnographic fieldwork was conducted in six residential care facilities for older persons in Sweden, several hours each week, during day and evening shifts, between January 2010 and June 2011, and from May 2014 to June 2015. A combination of participant observation and video-recordings was used to generate comprehensive insight into the overall routines per setting. For this chapter, field notes and audio-/video-recordings at three care units in two residential care facilities are used. One is a somatic unit hosting residents—the primary challenges lie in the area of mobility (dementia symptoms for some develop after admission). Two are dementia units hosting residents with neurological challenges. The observations presented in this chapter are based on 72 diaries of field notes and approximately 30 hours of video documentation of staff-resident interaction.

Participants who figure in the examples analyzed are four residents in their eighties (three females and one male under the pseudonyms Adila, Minna, Siri, and Ove), and five care workers (under the pseudonyms Medina, Stina, Anna, Moa, and Ivan). Minna, Siri, and Ove are diagnosed with Alzheimer's disease and are residents at dementia units. They are in the intermediate stages of the disease and receive help with their daily hygiene. Minna and Siri walk with trolleys (i.e., walkers), while Ove walks without an aiding device. Adila, who is wheelchair bound, is an Arabic-speaking resident living at a somatic unit. She immigrated to Sweden from Syria during old age. Whereas Adila and Siri have lived at the care facility for several years, Minna and Ove are rather new admittances.

Audio data have been transcribed according to conversation analytical principles (Ochs, Schegloff, & Thompson, 1996). Drawings illustrate bodily conduct. Embodied actions are transcribed according to conventions developed by Mondada (2014), see annotations presented in Chapter 1. Conversational video-recorded data in Arabic have been transcribed and then translated into Swedish by a proficient Arabic speaker. Translations from Swedish into English were made by the researcher and proofread by a Swedish-speaking, English native speaker. Each Swedish utterance is given an English translation in italics beneath it. Translations of Swedish into English are meant to be comprehensible, albeit not always altogether idiomatic.

Ethical Considerations

Data were collected in accordance with ethical guidelines established by the Swedish Research Council, and approved by a Regional Committee for Research Ethics (Dnr 2009-2003-31; Dnr 2013/2211-31).

All care workers and residents in the study gave consent to participate. The staff, residents, and their relatives were informed about the aims of the study and about their rights as participants by means of a letter and in personal encounters with the researchers who conducted the data collection. The Arabic-speaking resident received information about the project in her language. During the observations and recordings, researchers were on alert for any signs of the residents' unwillingness to be observed or recorded. All names have been changed to pseudonyms in the transcripts.

The Ambiguous Space of the Bathroom

While Extract 1 casts light on the unclear boundary between public and private that signifies the very nature of the care facility, in this section, I focus specifically on bathroom interactions, through which care workers negotiate their presence in this ambiguous space. The bathroom, whether in a person's ordinary home or in a resident's room at a care facility, is a place associated with intimacy and the primary care of bodies. It is a dedicated space relatively hidden from strangers, where private matters such as bathing, washing, and bodily excreting are accomplished. In a person's home, these activities are commonly done alone or in the company of close intimates (cf. Twigg, 1999, 2000). Any disability necessitating intimate care involves transgressing customary social rules concerning privacy. Within the care unit, the private territory of the individual then becomes the workplace of another; thus, trespassing on and reordering the divisions between public and private.

In a residential care facility, the bathroom is the place where the basic work of washing bodies takes place. As noted by Twigg (2000, p. 145) and demonstrated in ethnographic studies (Grainger, 1993; Jansson & Plejert, 2014; Plejert, Jansson, & Yazdanpanah, 2014), bodywork in care may involve embarrassing or painful procedures. Lee-Treweek (1994) shows how these aspects of care have to be managed spatially by being confined to the privacy of back bedrooms and bathrooms of the institution in order to present older persons clean and dressed in communal areas.

Examples analyzed in this section are drawn from morning care sessions at two different dementia units. In all examples, residents receive help with intimate care of the body (e.g., undressing, showering and massaging the body with lotion). Previous studies have highlighted some of the potential challenges associated with the task of assisting residents with intimate care and report on methods that can be used to minimize residents' opposition (Heinemann, 2009; Jansson & Plejert, 2014; Plejert et al., 2014; Yazdanpanah & Plejert, 2017). The role of humor (Heinemann, 2009) and body movement has been emphasized as crucial resources (Yazdanpanah & Plejert, 2017). The extracts below attend to care workers' use of bodily conduct to maintain an aspect of spatial privacy for residents during these care activities.

Maintaining Spatial Privacy

Care workers in Twigg's (1999) study report they would deliberately exit the bathroom and wait in the hall while clients bathed. This way of consciously maintaining an aspect of spatial privacy for the client does not occur in my data. One reason could be that the residents in my study, due to physical and cognitive impairment, require more assistance with the care activity. One reason might be that showering is a more 'advanced' activity to perform compared to sitting in a bath. While residents were put in shower chairs, the risk that they might fall remained. Additionally, maneuvering the shower tube (e.g., hose) requires finely tuned, coordinated movements, a procedure that was rarely left to residents.

Since care workers in my study could only leave residents out of sight momentarily, they only had at their disposal the area of the bathroom itself and, in many cases, the shower cabin to maintain a certain degree of privacy for residents. One strategy commonly observed among the care workers was to hand over the soap to residents and encourage them to wash their own bodies. During which, the care worker handled the maneuvering of the shower tube while keeping a certain corporeal distance from the resident, thus allowing the resident to retain some of the sense of being alone. Extract 2 exemplifies such a strategy. The extract involves a male resident (R) Ove and a female care worker (CW) Moa. Ove was sometimes perceived by the care workers as a 'difficult' resident, particularly when it came to showering. They reported that he often refused to shower or reacted with challenging behavior. In this particular case, the resident knew the care worker and, as will be shown, the two got along rather well. The camera is directed toward the care worker. The resident, who is hidden behind the shower curtain, is out of camera shot. The curtain is half open, so it is possible to see the care worker's actions. The extract begins a few minutes into the shower when Moa is rinsing shampoo from Ove's hair.

Extract 2: Moa is rinsing the shampoo from Ove's hair with the shower tube

01.	Ove:	ho ho
	(R)	*ho ho*
02.	Moa:	Δ*bends down; rinses the shampoo from O's*
	(CW)	*hair----->*
		#fig. 11.2
03.	Moa:	du ser ut som en riktig sportdykare
		you look like a real sport diver
		--

04.		(10.0) ((*M rinses the shampoo*))
05.	Moa:	varsågod Ove (.) nu får du tvätta
		dej
		here you go Ove (.) *now you can wash*
		yourself
		--
		-----Δ
06.		så sköter jag vattnet
		I will take care of the water then
		Δ*raises body*--------Δ
		#fig.11.3
07.	Ove:	(ja)ha
		well yes
08.	Moa:	m:↑m
		m:↑m
09.		(4.5) ((*showering goes on*))
10.	Moa:	Δ*takes a step aside; gazes downward*
		----------------------------------->>
		#fig. 11.4
11.		(2.0) ((*showering goes on*))

12.	Moa:	kan man se som lite morrongymnastik sam- tidigt (.) *you can regard this as some morning exer- cise at the same (.)*
13.		eller h↑u:r. *time can't you*
14.	Ove :	ja [man får göra de ja (.) (man) får stå på h(h)änderna *yes you may do that yea (.) (you) may stand on your hands*
15.	Moa:	[j¿:a *[y:ea*
16.		he he [he he he ((*laughter*))
17.	Ove:	[hi hi hi hi .h he he he he .h (.) ja:a ((*laughter*)) (.) *ye:a*

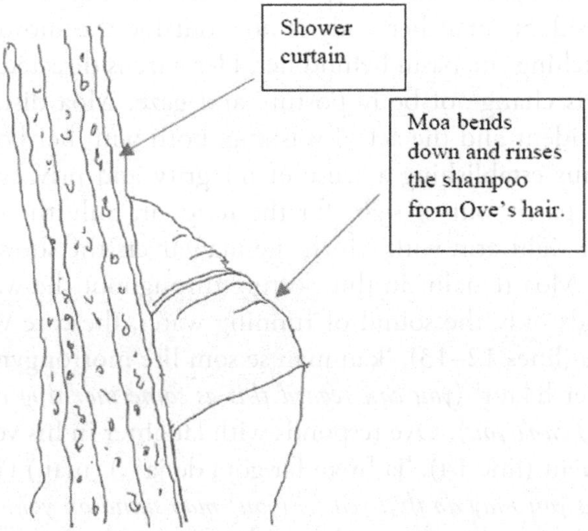

Fig. 11.2 Ove behind shower curtain; Moa rinses shampoo from Ove's hair (*Source* Author)

In line 02, Moa bends down and rinses shampoo from the resident's hair (Fig. 11.2). She is now inside the shower cabinet and close to the resident's body. At this moment, when the water is raining down from Ove's head, Moa likens him to a sport diver. This is a delicate moment in the shower activity as something is being done to the resident (Jansson & Plejert, 2014; Twigg, 2000). The care worker controls this task; the resident is not allocated any active part of the task. Still, the way the resident is portrayed as a sport diver invokes a masculine and vigorous identity, and dispels any potential unpleasant or threatening experience of the hair wash. Having finished the hair wash, Moa leaves the washing of the body to the resident (lines 05–06), 'varsågod Ove (.) nu får du tvätta dej så sköter jag vattnet' (h*ere you go Ove (.) now you can wash yourself I will take care of the water then*). She raises, withdraws her left hand, and maneuvers the shower tube with her right hand (Fig. 11.3). In line 10, she takes a step aside in an outward direction from the cabinet area (Fig. 11.4), withdrawing herself physically from the resident. Half her body is now outside the shower cabin, her left arm touching the basin behind her. Her gaze is directed downwards. Through this change of body posture and gaze, Moa distances herself from the resident and the act of washing, both with her body and with her gaze, thus establishing a sense of integrity and privacy for the resident. Now partly out of sight for the resident, only the care worker's face and her right arm with which she maneuvers the shower tube is in Ove's sight. Moa remains in this posture throughout the washing. After seven seconds only the sound of running water, the care worker introduces a joke (lines 12–13), 'kan man se som lite morrongymnastik samtidigt (.) eller h↑u:r' (*you can regard this as some morning exercise at the same time (.) can't you*). Ove responds with laughter in his voice, conveying amusement (line 14), 'ja [man får göra de ja (.) (man) får stå på h(h) änderna' (*yes you may do that yea (.) (you) may stand on your hands*). This response indicates that Ove endorses the care worker's jocular categorization of the shower as morning exercise. Moa starts laughing, and Ove overlaps with laughter resulting in joint laughter (lines 16–17).

In Extract 2, body posture and gaze direction stand out as prominent resources for the management of spatial privacy. The jocular tone dispels

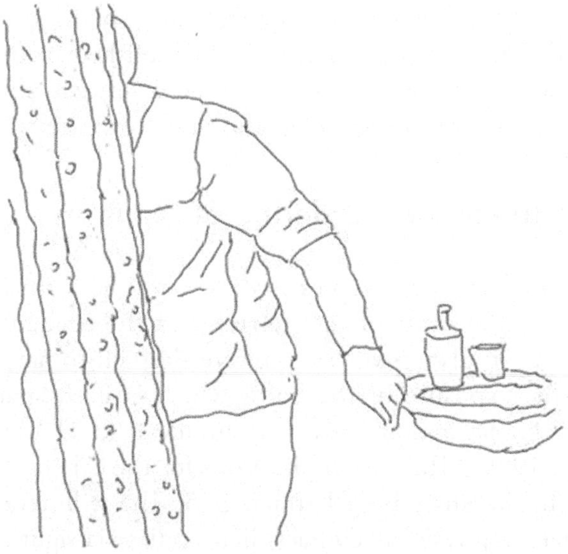

Fig. 11.3 Moa attending to water (*Source* Author)

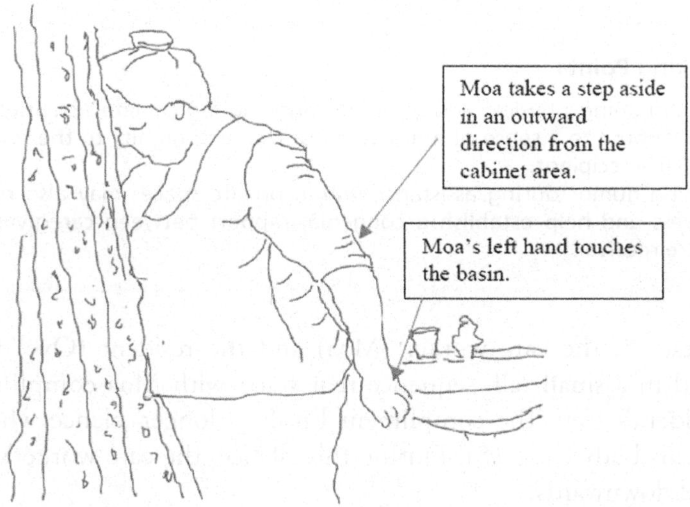

Fig. 11.4 Moa stepping aside (*Source* Author)

potential aspects of embarrassment invoked by physical exposure. The washing of the body, a private matter accomplished in the presence of another, is thereby cast as a moment of shared amusement. All this contributes to preserving some sense of autonomy for the resident.

Managing the Spatial Ordering of the Body

Help with the shower task represents not only the intrusion of professional care into the most private territory of the resident's apartment, the bathroom, it also involves transgressing customary social rules concerning the exposure of the body, which is itself spatially ordered according to gradations of privacy (Jourard, 1966; Jourard & Rubin, 1968; Twigg, 1999). This has implications for the care encounter, which is discussed in the analysis of Extracts 3–5. The willingness of persons to allow others to physically contact their bodies via sight and touch is a function of the closeness of the relationship. Extracts 3–5 illustrate how care workers manage this spatial ordering of the body during intimate care.

Thinking Points

1. Maintaining physical and visual distance during private activities may contribute to a sense of autonomy, control, and dignity to the resident or care recipient.
2. Using humor during assistance within private spaces may also relieve stress and help establish a congenial rapport between caregiver and care receiver.

In Extract 3, the care worker (Moa) and the resident (Ove) become involved in a small talk sequence that starts with Moa complimenting the resident's feet. The compliment breaks a longer silence while Ove washes his body (line 18). During this silence, the care worker's gaze is directed downwards.

Extract 3: Moa and Ove continuation of shower

18.		(2.0) ((*M holds the shower tube; gazes downwards*))
19.	Moa:	vilka fina fötter du har *what nice feet you have* Δ*looks down at O's feet; turns body aside*-----> #fig. 11.5
20.		(0.5)
21.	Ove:	ja verkligen *yes really*
	moa:	----------→
22.	Moa:	ja jättefina *yes really nice* --------------→
23.	Ove:	ja:a de var ju vänligt *yeah that was really kind*
	moa:	----------------------------Δ
24.	Moa:	dom var (xx) dom var snygga att titta på *they are* (xx) *nice to look at* #fig. 11.6
25.		(0.7)
26.	Ove:	he he he ((*laughter*))
	moa:	----------Δ
27.	Moa:	faktiskt *really*
	moa:	Δ*bends her upper body down*------------>> #fig. 11.7
28.		(2.0) ((*showering goes on*))
29.	Moa:	man ska vara rädd om fötterna *you should take care of your feet*
30.	Ove:	javisst ska man de *yes indeed you should*
31.	Moa:	m:: (.) dom ska bära en he:la livet *m::* (.) *they should carry you your whole life*
32.	Ove:	oj oj oj *oh oh oh*
33.	Moa:	ja::↑a *ye::a*
34.	Ove:	å dom sparkar på en å *and they kick you also*
35.	Moa:	ja:::[de gö'rom *ye::* [*a they do*
36.	Ove:	[he he he he he ((*laughter*))

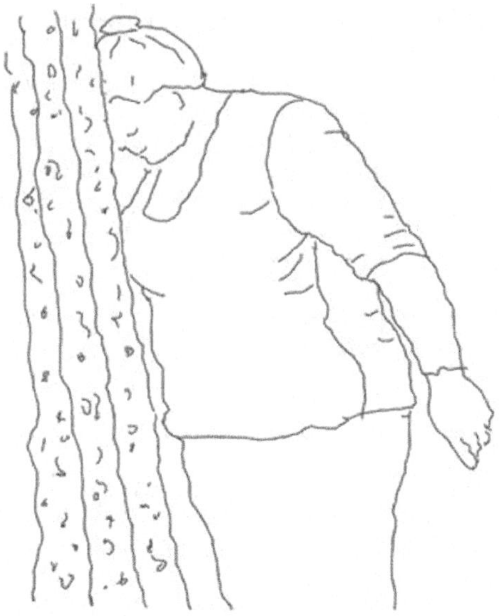

Fig. 11.5 Moa gazes downward (*Source* Author)

In line 19, Moa looks down and compliments Ove's feet with a praise assessment (Fig. 11.5), 'vilka fina fötter du har' (what nice feet you have). Ove makes the same evaluation and agrees, 'ja verkligen' (*yes really*). In response, Moa proffers a second assessment, 'ja jättefina' (*yes really nice*). The resident shows appreciation for the compliment, 'ja:a de var ju vänligt' (*yes that was really kind*). In line 24, the care worker turns her body aside and withdraws the shower tube (Fig. 11.6), while offering more praise, 'dom var snygga att titta på' (*they are nice to look at*). The resident responds with amused laughter (line 26). In line 27, Moa bends down and asserts her positive evaluation, 'faktiskt' (*really*). She bends her upper body down so as to come closer to Ove's feet with her gaze (Fig. 11.7). This reciprocal praising of the resident's feet is followed by a small talk sequence focusing on feet in general (lines 29–35).

As the interaction in this extract occurs during the washing of the body, the care worker, assisting the resident when needed, runs the risk of being cast into the role of an observer, a role that might be sensitive given the resident's nakedness. The small talk sequence about Ove's feet

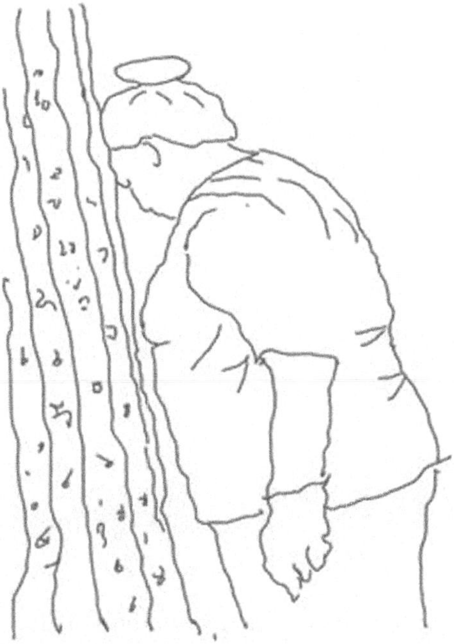

Fig. 11.6 Moa looking down (*Source* Author)

and about feet in general break a potentially embarrassing silence. As such, the reciprocal praising and the way the participants agree with one another help to create and reinforce social affiliation (Pomerantz, 1984). In addition, it helps the participants avoid focusing on sensitive parts of the body.

Thinking Points

1. Small talk during assistance in private spaces during private acts such as showering may alleviate the care receiver's embarrassment or feelings of intrusion.
2. Through careful diversion of body and gaze, the caregiver may circumvent awkwardness that may occur in self and in the care receiver.

The next example (Extract 4) involves a male care worker Ivan and a female resident Minna. The example is drawn from an audio recording

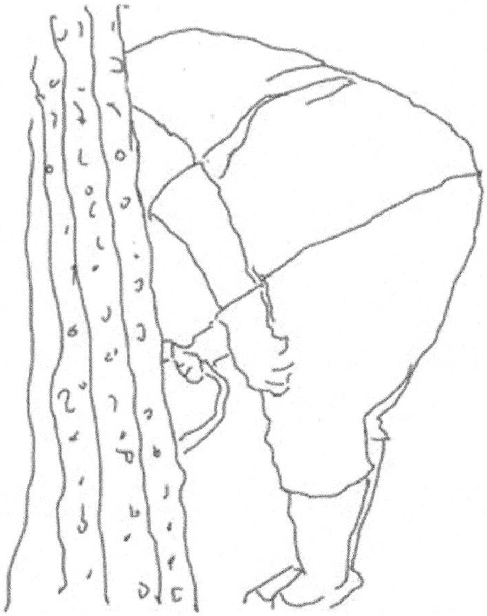

Fig. 11.7 Moa gazing at Ove's feet (*Source* Author)

during a morning activity in the resident's bathroom, as the resident is undressed and prepared to shower. In this example, the locus of shared attention is the resident's shoes. From the care worker's procedural talk preceding the extract, the task of undressing, except for the shoes, has been carried out when the extract begins.

Extract 4: Ivan and Minna focus on shoes

01.	Ivan: (CW)	så: (.) nu får du sätta dej *there (.) now you can sit down*
02.		(18.0) ((*scratch sound*))
03.	Ivan:	vilka fina skor du har Minna *what nice shoes you have Minna*
04.	Minna: (R)	m:
05.	Ivan:	ja::. var har du köpte dom? *yea where did you buy them*
06.	Minna:	de var länge sen *it was a long time ago*

07.	Ivan:	de var [länge sen
		it was a [long time ago
08.	Minna:	[de vet ja'nte
		[I don't know
09.	Ivan:	ja:::. men dom e jättefina
		ye:::a but they are really nice
10.	Minna:	ja de e'rom
		yes they are
11.		(3.0)
12.	Minna:	ja måste ha strumpor på mej
		I must have socks on
13.	Ivan:	ja de ska du få (.) men ja tänkte bara
		yes you will (.) but I only thought
14.		ta av den hära (.) d[å får du nya kläder
		I'd take off this one (.) then you will have new clothes
15.	Minna:	[å: då fryser ja ihjäl ännu mera
		[oh then I will die of cold even more
16.	Ivan:	ja f[örstår de (.) ja ska stänga dörren
		I understand that (.) I will lock the door
17.	Minna:	[å va hemskt
		[oh how awful
18.		(2.0)
19.	Minna:	de e så kallt
		it's so cold
20.	Ivan:	ja:
		yea
21.	Minna:	de e så kallt (.) å: de e som de var ute
		it's so cold (.) oh it's as if we were outdoors

Ivan begins by asking the resident to sit down on the shower chair. Minna has just been undressed, her nightdress and her trousers taken off. The vulnerable parts of the resident's body are thus exposed; only the feet are covered. The compliment in line 3 breaks a rather long silence, when Ivan then takes off the resident's shoes. The small talk about Minna's shoes helps the care worker defuse tensions and mitigate the experience of being exposed. In addition, it helps the care worker avoid talking about the more private parts of the body. In line 12, Minna objects to having her socks taken off, the only clothing sheltering her body. When Ivan suggests removing the socks, despite Minna's expressed desire to have them on, 'men ja tänkte bara ta av den härä' (*but I only thought I'd take off this one*), the resident escalates her opposition with an extreme case formulation (Pomerantz, 1986), 'å: då fryser ja ihjäl ännu mera' (*oh then* ***I will die*** *of cold even more* [emphasis added]). Despite Ivan's negotiations, the continuation of the interaction, marked by opposition and complaining, embodies the vulnerability that frames the care encounter.

Thinking Points

1. Complaints by care recipient may, indeed, be diversions from the discomfort of the loss of privacy.
2. Co-participants may consider acknowledging such complaints as a way to maintain the care recipient's dignity and relieve tensions arising from the necessity of occupying the care recipient's private space.

In Extract 5, which involves Siri and Anna, neutral areas of the body—the back and the hands (Jourard, 1966)—are emphasized. Siri has had a shower and is presently sitting in a chair in the hall outside the bathroom (see Fig. 11.8). Prior to this extract, Anna has towel dried the resident's back.

Extract 5: Siri and Anna focus on neutral areas of the body

```
01.  Anna:    (2.0)+massages Siri's back with lotion------>
     (CW)
02.  Siri:    å va skönt de va på ryggen
     (R)      oh that felt good    on my back
     anna:    ---------------------------------+
03.  Anna:    m:m (.) °ja ska ta°
              m:m (.) I'll take
              +moves hand to Siri's arm+
04.           (1.5) ((A massages Siri's left underarm with
               lotion))
05.  Anna:    va fin du e på arm- händerna nu
              your arm- hands look really nice now
              +massages Siri's left hand; caresses it with her
              index finger-------------------+
              #fig.11.8
06.  Anna:    +massages Siri's hand----->
```

```
07.  Siri:   Ja
     anna:   yes
             ---+
08.  Anna:   nu e'ru inte alls så där narig som du var ett tag
             now you are not at all as chapped as you were
             +massages Siri's left arm---------------------->
09.          ------+(0.5)
10.  Siri:   ja ja  (.) jo ja e rädd om de för att ja [spe-
             yea yea (.) well I take care of them since I pla-
     anna:   +massages Siri's left hand----------------->
11.  Anna:                                            [ja:
                                                      [ye:a
12.  Siri:   spelar ju så att
             play so
13.  anna:   ----------------+(0.5)
14.  Siri:   [man kan
             [one can
     anna:   +massages Siri's left arm---->
15.  Anna:   [man måste va rädd om dej
             [someone needs to take care of you
             ------------------------>
16.  Siri:   använda händerna till de
             use your hands for that
     anna:   ----------------------+
17.  Anna:   precis
             exactly
             +moves her hand to Siri's back----->>
```

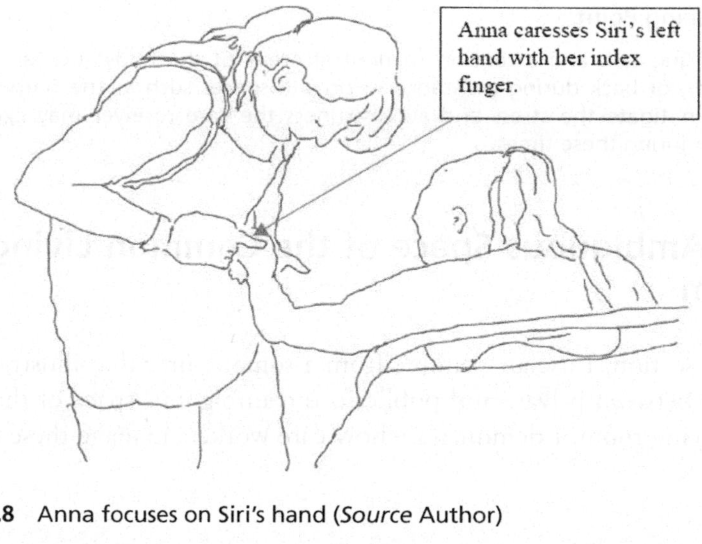

Fig. 11.8 Anna focuses on Siri's hand (*Source* Author)

Anna is applying lotion to Siri's body with gentle massaging movements, sheltering Siri's back with a towel (line 01). The resident assesses this as comfortable and nice (line 02). Anna continues rubbing the resident's left arm, and when she arrives at Siri's hand, she bends her upper body down so as to come closer to the resident's hand with her gaze (Fig. 11.8). While caressing Siri's left hand, she compliments the quality of her hands. Anna then moves to Siri's arm. She holds the resident's hand as she massages the arm with lotion, remarking that her hands are no longer chapped (lines 08–09). Anna's compliment opens up a conversation about Siri's hands and the role of hands. As Anna continues massaging the resident's hands and arms (lines 10–17), Siri indicates that she takes care of her hands, emphasizing she plays the piano, which Anna approves.

By highlighting Siri's hand—focusing her gaze and complimenting it—the care worker minimizes attention to the resident's more private parts of the body. In compliance, the resident makes her hand accessible to visual and tactual contact. This mutual orientation of the participants' bodies toward the region of the resident's body they are discussing and working with creates a public focus of attention, allowing the private to remain private.

Thinking Point

Diverting talk and attention to neutral areas of the body such as feet, hands, or back during assistance in private spaces such as the bathroom may mitigate the stress and awkwardness the care receiver may experience during these times.

The Ambiguous Space of the Common Living Room

In this section, I use an example from a somatic unit that illustrates the clashes between private and public in the ambiguous space of the common living room. I demonstrate how care workers manage these clashes

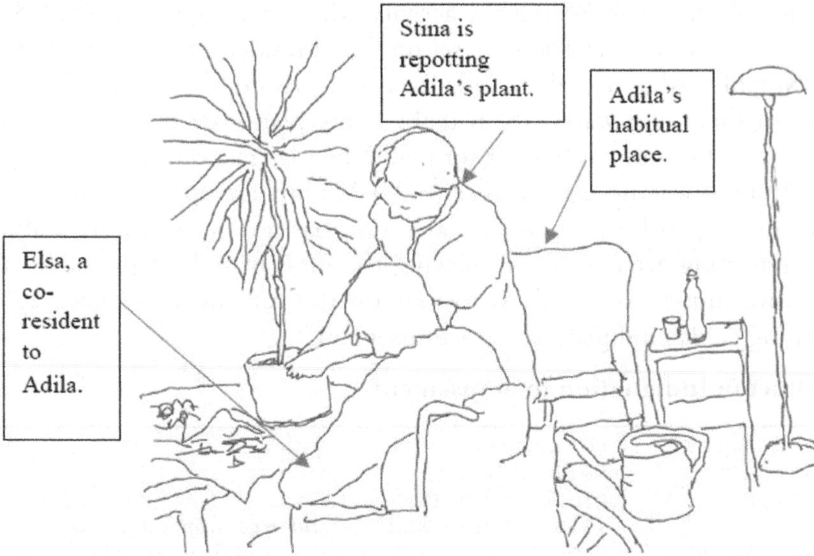
Stina is
repotting
Adila's plant.
Adila's
habitual
place.
Elsa, a
co-
resident
to
Adila.

Fig. 11.9 Repotting activity (*Source* Author)

that emanate from unclear boundaries. The example is divided into two extracts, 6 and 7.

One theme evolving from the empirical data in the study of Hauge and Heggen (2008, p. 464) was the lack of social relationships between the residents: '[T]he residents live their everyday lives in a room with ambiguous boundaries and have hardly any social relationships among themselves'. Those residents who were mobile typically withdraw to their own rooms to maintain a degree of privacy. Adila, by contrast, has created for herself a private sphere in a corner of the common living room, spending up to 10 hours a day here, making it her habitual place. Adila usually sits in an armchair with a small table beside her where she has her afternoon coffee (see Fig. 11.9). On the table she has a bottle with water she uses for watering the potted plants. Consequently, the care staff also considered this corner Adila's space.

Extracts 6 and 7 are drawn from an episode in which a care worker (CW) Stina is engaged in repotting the plants in Adila's habitual place (see Fig. 11.9). Elsa, a Swedish-speaking co-resident of Adila's, is sitting in her wheelchair watching the activity. The repotting was scheduled by the care staff as a social activity set up for all residents at the care unit.

Notably, Adila regards the plants as her private belongings: she takes care of them and waters them daily. Some plants are from exotic fruit seeds that her son has bought for her. When Extract 6 begins, Adila and an Arabic-speaking care worker (CW) Medina are approaching. Adila, having napped for an hour in her room, has not been informed about the repotting activity. Upon viewing the mess of soil on the table, she becomes upset. The analysis focuses on the care workers' practices in turning Adila's indignation into amusement.

Extract 6: Indignation to amusement

```
01.   Stina:     hej Adila.
      (CW)       hello Adila.
                 ¤looks at Adila----->
02.              (0.5)((Adila and Medina are approaching))
03.   Medina:    shoufi        [shou aam ya´amloulek bi
      (CW)       look what they are doing with
      stina:     ----------------------------------------
04.   Stina:                   [he::j.
                               [hello
                               -------¤
05.   Medina:    zara'tek shoufi
                 your plants look
06.              (1.1) ((Stina leaves hold of the plant;
07.              steps forward on the floor gazing at A))
08.   Adila:     shou dakhalltili bi zar´ati
      (R)        what do you put in my plants
                 *makes a hand point*
      stina:     ¤moves the tray with soil aside---¤(0.5)
      medina:    +smiles------------------------+
09.   Medina:    hhhhh(.)£va g¿ö:r du me mi- he(h)nnes£
                  h[hhhhhhh
                 what are you doing with m- her
      stina:     ¤smiles and looks at
                  Adila-------------------->>
                 #fig. 11.10
```

When Adila approaches, Stina looks up from the plant and greets her (line 01). In line 03, Medina bids for Adila's attention with a smile, 'shoufi shou[aam ya´amloulek bi zara'tek shoufi' (*look what they are*

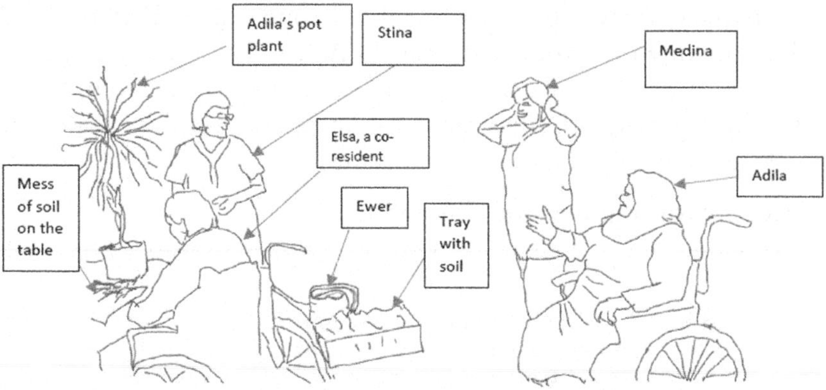

Fig. 11.10 Repotting configuration of participants (*Source* Author)

doing with your plants look). The fact that Medina assesses the event as something remarkable is corroborated by the fact that she recycles the verb 'shoufi' (*look*) and refers to the plants as Adila's by use of the Arabic possessive suffix /tek/(*your*) in 'zara'tek' (*plants- your*). Arriving where the repotting is occurring, Medina turns away from Adila and places her wheelchair in a position right in front of Stina, who is standing at the table with the plants. Stina also makes arrangements to create space for Adila and invites her to participate. She greets Adila, steps forward and moves aside a tray with soil. The care workers' bid for attention encourages Adila to display emotion. In line 08, seeing her potted plants, the mess of soil, and empty pots on the table, she responds with indignation. Pointing with her hand and gazing at the plants on the table, she issues a question in Arabic with an indignant voice, 'shou dakhalltili bi zar'ati' (*what do you put in my plants*), thus assessing the local scene as an unexpected and accountable event (Fig. 11.10). Following Adila's reaction, Medina starts laughing (line 09). She turns her gaze to Stina and voices Adila's Arabic speech in Swedish for her. Medina's rendition of Adila's response cry (Goffman, 1981) is produced with a high pitch and within-speech laugh particles conveying a stance of amusement, '£va g¿ö:r du me mi- he(h)nnes£ h[hhhhhhh' (*what are you doing with m- her*). This change of framing (Goffman, 1974) constitutes a shift in affective stance compared to Adila's prior talk, a switch from serious indignation to agreeable surprise and amusement.

In Extract 7, which follows eight seconds after Extract 6, the Arabic-speaking care workers explain to Adila what Stina is doing with her plants. I demonstrate how the care workers cast the complainable event, the repotting of Adila's plants, as an activity worthy of praise and how Adila eventually aligns with this frame.

Extract 7: Working towards alignment

20.		((*8 seconds of recording; Adila displays indignation*))
21.	Medina:	aam behoutollon trab ahmar
		they are putting red soil into them
		+*points at the table with pot plants*+
22.		>ja sa dom [behöver< jo::rd
		I said they need soil
		+gazes at Stina-------------+
23.	Stina:	[ny: j¿o::rd.
		[*new soil*
		¤*gesticulates; looks at Adila*¤
24.	Stina:	ja::a (.) ja:: (.) (xx)
		yea (.) *yea* (.) (*xx*)
		¤*looks at Adila*--------->>
		Δ*smiles; tilts head aside*Δ
25.	Medina:	lazemlen trab ahmar jd¿id, (.) hadjeh.
		they need new red soil lady
		+*points at the tray with soil on the floor*+
26.	Adila:	bra[:
		good
		nods and smiles
		ø*gazes at Stina*--------->>
27.	Stina:	[hon tycker de e henne [s blommor
		[*she thinks that they're* [*her flowers*
28.	Medina:	[bra:vo (.)
		[*bravo* (.)
	adila:	**smiles*----->>
29	Medina:	hon [tycker bra:↑vo
		she [*thinks bravo*
30.	Stina:	[hhhhahahhahahaha [hahahahahahaha ((*laughter*))
31.	Medina:	[hahahaha ((*laughter*))

Medina explains to Adila in Arabic that they are adding fresh soil, 'aam behoutollon trab ahmar' (*they are putting red soil into them*). By emphasizing the initial syllable while making an extended hand pointing at the table with potted plants, she describes the event as something worthy of attention. She then turns to Stina and reports in Swedish what she just said in Arabic to Adila (line 22), '>ja sa dom behöver<jo::rd' (*I said they need soil*). Stina looks at Adila and highlights the material, the new soil, in Swedish, '[ny: j¿o::rd'. (*new soil*). While pointing at the tray with soil on the floor, Medina rephrases in Arabic the information about new soil that they have collectively emphasized in the preceding talk in Swedish, 'lezemlen trab ahmar jd¿id, (.) hadjeh'. (*they need new red soil lady*). In response, Adila evaluates the repotting as worthy of appreciation with the assessment term 'bra:' (*good*) in Swedish. She holds her gaze on Stina while smiling and nodding. In line 27, Stina emphatically aligns with Adila's display of indignation in previous turns by confirming the fact that Adila regards the plants as hers, 'hon tycker de e henne[s blommor' (*she thinks that they're her flowers*). In overlap, Medina rephrases Adila's assessment turn in Swedish with an upgrade, 'bravo' (*bravo*) that she subsequently recycles, 'hon tycker bra:↑vo' (*she thinks bravo*). Stina responds with a stream of laughter (line 30) and Medina overlaps with further laughter resulting in laughing together.

The grounds for Adila's indignation in this example may appear unresolvable. It may well be the case that Adila's having a specific habitual place in the common living room has created a sense of home for her and an 'attachment to space' (cf. Falk et al., 2012, p. 1003). As viewed from an institutional perspective, the corner where Adila has her habitual place is a public space and hence no one's private sphere. Even though Adila takes care of the potted plants as if they were hers, they are no one's private belongings. Most have been bought by the institution as part of the public decoration of the care facility. Potted plants can, however, be seen as typical symbols that mark a private living room. In her challenging question to the care workers (Extract 6, line 08), 'shou dakhalltili bi zar'ati' (*what do you put in my plants*), Adila refers to the plants as hers. Also the care workers refer to the plants as Adila's (see Extract 6, line 05 and Extract 7, line 27). This is their way of aligning with Alina's ownership of the plants and the possible transgression she experienced when not informed about the repotting of her plants.

Summary

In this chapter, I have presented observations on care workers' and residents' negotiation of public and private in residential care facilities for older people in Sweden. From the data, I account for the methods that care workers adopt to order space in a way that maintains a sense of privacy and dignity for the resident. I demonstrate (1) how care workers negotiate their presence in the ambiguous space of bathrooms; (2) how they manage the resident's body according to gradations of privacy. I show that body posture, gaze direction, and reciprocal praising stand out as prominent resources for this management. The analysis attests to how the participants mutually orient to the neutral parts of the body, such as the feet and the hands. Focus on the neutral regions of the body (or with accessories such as the shoes in Extract 4) allows both care workers to avoid contact with more private parts and all participants to avoid naming these parts with direct language, strategies that work to negotiate body taboos. Extracts 6 and 7 focus on the clashes between private and public in the ambiguous space of the common living room and how care workers manage these clashes, largely by emphatically aligning with the residents' views.

Practical Implications

The findings suggest that despite unavoidable clashes between private and public spheres in the ambiguous space of care facilities, care workers possess methods to manage these clashes. What particularly stands out in all data extracts is the way the care workers cast an embarrassing situation as a moment of amusement through affect-regulating practices. Additional ways to negotiate the private and public ambiguity of space required in all caregiving settings are presented in the Practical Highlights section below.

Practical Highlights

1. Fine-grained verbal and nonverbal interactional moves work to negotiate privacy boundaries—physical and visual.
2. Bodily posture and gaze direction are prominent resources for the management of spatial privacy in the private territory of the resident's bathroom.
3. Casting potential breaches into private spaces or activities as a moment of shared amusement dispels potential aspects of embarrassment.
4. Mutual orientation to the neutral parts of the body, such as the resident's feet, hands, and back may help maintain customary social rules concerning the exposure of the body.
5. Small talk, gaze direction, and reciprocal praise are examples of methods.
6. Unavoidable clashes between public and private in the ambiguous space can be managed through affect-regulating practices (e.g., shared laughter, a jocular tone) and through emphatically aligning with the resident's view.

References

Allan, G., & Crow, G. (1989). Introduction. In G. Allan & G. Crow (Eds.), *Home and family: Creating the domestic sphere* (pp. 1–13). Houndmills, Basingstoke, Hampshire, UK and New York, NY: Palgrave.

Douglas, M. (1991). The idea of a home: A kind of space. *Social Research, 58*(1), 287–307.

Falk, H., Wijk, H., & Falk, K. (2012). A sense of home in residential care. *Scandinavian Journal of Caring Sciences, 27*(4), 999–1009.

Goffman, E. (1961). *Asylum: Essays of the social situations of mental patients and other inmates*. New York, NY: Doubleday.

Goffman, E. (1974). *Frame analysis: An essay on the organization of experience*. Boston, MA: Northeastern University Press.

Goffman, E. (1981). *Forms of talk*. Oxford, UK: Basil Blackwell.

Grainger, K. (1993). "That's a lovely bath dear": Reality construction in the discourse of elderly care. *Journal of Aging Studies, 7*(3), 247–262.

Hammersley, M., & Atkinson, P. (Eds.). (2007). *Ethnography: Principles in practice* (3rd ed.). London, UK: Routledge.

Hauge, S., & Heggen, K. (2008). The nursing home as a home: A field study of residents' daily life in the common living room. *Journal of Clinical Nursing, 17*(4), 460–467.
Heinemann, T. (2009). Participation and exclusion in third party complaints. *Journal of Pragmatics, 41*(12), 2435–2451.
Heinemann, T. (2011). From home to institution: Roles, relations and the loss of autonomy in the care of old people in Denmark. In P. Backhaus (Ed.), *Communication in elderly care: Cross-cultural perspectives* (pp. 90–111). London, UK and New York, NY: Continuum.
Higgins, J. (1989). Home and institutions. In G. Allan & G. Crow (Eds.), *Home and family: Creating the domestic sphere* (pp. 159–173). Houndmills, Basingstoke, Hampshire, UK and New York, NY: Palgrave.
Higgins, I. (1998). Pearls, pith and provocation: Reflections on conducting qualitative research with elderly people. *Qualitative Health Research, 8*(6), 858–866.
Jansson, G. (2016). "You're doing everything just fine": Praise in residential care settings. *Discourse Studies, 18*(1), 64–86.
Jansson, G., & Nikolaidou, Z. (2013). Work-identity in ethnographic research: Developing field roles in a demanding workplace setting. *International Journal of Qualitative Methods, 12*(1), 152–167.
Jansson, G., & Plejert, C. (2014). Taking a shower: Managing a potentially imposing activity in dementia care. *Journal of Interactional Research in Communication Disorders, 5*(1), 27–62.
Jansson, G., Wadensjö, C., & Plejert, C. (2017). Managing complaints in multilingual care encounters. *Multilingua*. https://doi.org/10.1515/MULTI-2016-0043.
Jourard, S. M. (1966). An exploratory study of body-accessibility. *British Journal of Social and Clinical Psychology, 5*(3), 221–231.
Jourard, S. M., & Rubin, J. E. (1968). Self-disclosure and touching: A study of two modes of interpersonal encounter and their inter-relation. *Journal of Humanistic Psychology, 8*(1), 39–48.
Lee-Treweek, G. (1994). Bedroom abuse: The hidden work in a nursing home. *Generations Review, 4*(1), 2–4.
Lee-Treweek, G. (1998). Normality is hard work: Trade unions and the politics of community care. *Work, Employment & Society, 12*(2), 388–389.
Makoni, S., & Grainger, K. (2002). Comparative gerontolinguistics: Characterizing discourses in caring institutions in South Africa and the United Kingdom. *Journal of Social Issues, 58*(4), 805–824.

Mondada, L. (2014). *Conventions for multimodal transcriptions.* Retrieved from https://franz.unibas.ch/fileadmin/franz/user_upload/redaktion/Mondada_conv_multimodality.pdf

Nussbaum, J. F. (1993). The communication impact of institutionalization for the elderly: The admission process. *Journal of Aging Studies, 7*(3), 237–246.

Ochs, E., Schegloff, E. A., & Thompson, S. A. (1996). *Interaction and grammar.* Cambridge, UK: Cambridge University Press.

Plejert, C., Jansson, G., & Yazdanpanah, M. (2014). Response practices in multilingual interaction with an older Persian woman in a Swedish residential home. *Journal of Cross-Cultural Gerontology, 29*(1), 1–23.

Pomerantz, A. (1984). Agreeing and disagreeing with assessments: Some features of preferred/dispreferred turn shapes. In J. M. Atkinson & J. Heritage (Eds.), *Structures of social action. Studies in conversation analysis* (pp. 57–101). Cambridge, UK: Cambridge University Press.

Pomerantz, A. (1986). Extreme case formulations: A way of legitimizing claims. *Human Studies, 9,* 219–229.

Ridell, K. (2008). *Dansk-svenska samtal i praktiken. Språklig interatkion och ackommodation mellan äldre och vårdpersonal i Öresundsregionen.* [Danish-Swedish conversation in practice. Linguistic interaction and accommodation between the elderly and their caregivers in the Öresund region.] Skrifter utgivna av Institutionen för nordiska språk 76 vid Uppsala, SE: Uppsala Universitet.

Sidnell, J., & Stivers, T. (2013). *The handbook of conversation analysis.* West Sussex, UK: Wiley-Blackwell.

Twigg, J. (1999). The spatial ordering of care: Public and private in bathing support at home. *Sociology of Health & Illness, 21*(4), 381–400.

Twigg, J. (2000). *Bathing. The body and community care.* New York, NY and London, UK: Routledge.

Williams, K. N. (2011). Elderspeak in institutional care for older adults. In P. Backhaus (Ed.), *Communication in elderly care: Cross-cultural perspectives* (pp. 1–19). London, UK and New York, NY: Continuum.

Yazdanpanah, M., & Plejert, C. (2017). Accommodation practices in multilingual encounters in residential care in Sweden. In C. Plejert, C. Lindholm, & R. W. Shrauf (Eds.), *Multilingual interaction and dementia* (pp. 148–174). Bristol, UK: Multilingual Matters.

Recommended Readings

Falk, H., Wijk, H., & Falk, K. (2012). A sense of home in residential care. *Scandinavian Journal of Caring Sciences, 27*(4), 999–1009.

Jansson, G., & Plejert, C. (2014). Taking a shower: Managing a potentially imposing activity in dementia care. *Journal of Interactional Research in Communication Disorders, 5*(1), 27–62.

Twigg, J. (2000). *Bathing. The body and community care.* New York, NY and London, UK: Routledge.

Part III

Conclusion: Keeping the Conversation Going

12

Conclusion: Keeping the Conversation Going

Trini Stickle

What We Have Learned

As I reflected on the many conversations presented within each chapter and the nuanced observations on those conversations, I realized how critical the particular context was to understanding each. Any attempt to merely summarize the chapters and their highlights would run the risk of creating what seemed to be a detailed rulebook for successful conversation. Yet, no such rulebook exists. Many of the specific recommendations given in each chapter provide potential tools for successful interaction, tools best chosen depending on the particular task at hand, a task that may not fully be known until in the midst of conversation. Some general principles that emerge from this work and which may guide the selection of a specific tool are, however, worth bringing to the conversation.

T. Stickle (✉)
Western Kentucky University, Bowling Green, KY, USA
e-mail: trini.stickle@wku.edu

T. Stickle (ed.), *Learning from the Talk of Persons with Dementia*,
The Language of Mental Health, https://doi.org/10.1007/978-3-030-43977-4_12

Perhaps foremost among these principles is the need for careful and engaged listening. Careful, in that one must pay attention to the specific linguistic choices that a person with dementia makes, particularly as those choices may be used in unexpected ways (Chapter 5). Engaged, in that one must acknowledge through apt verbal and nonverbal cues that one is actively listening. In all cases, one must allow the person ample time to respond. Keep in mind that while you are listening, you could, occasionally, hear talk that is difficult to understand. As a result, you may be unsure how to respond. Simply acknowledging that you are still listening (through brief utterances like *mmm hmm*, *uh huh*, *right*, *yeah*) may be the best choice to keep some form of conversation going, while waiting for the possibility that (more) coherent talk emerges (Chapters 6 and 7).

Sometimes, before you can listen, you may have to encourage talk. In our day-to-day discourse, we use questions to this end. When talking with people who have dementia, however, questions, particularly of some forms, can oftentimes tax their memory and inject unnecessary difficulty into the conversation (Chapter 3). An alternative strategy would be to draw the person's attention to an interesting object within reach or sight (Chapters 8 and 9). One could ask questions about the object, but one could also simply comment, or give an assessment. The goal is to find something of interest to the person, something in the environment to stimulate talk. Give the person time; defer control; let the person with dementia share interests, knowledge, and concerns. Keep listening.

As you listen, be prepared for departures from expected interactional patterns. This can be difficult. The conventions and practices of talk can be deeply ingrained. When a person with dementia produces a linguistic construction or a social action (through language) that diverges from typical patterns, we can easily find ourselves frustrated, confused, or dismayed (Chapters 7 and 9). Patience and empathy *are* in order; correction may not always be. Remain aware of the nature of the disorder, with progressive declines in memory and communication abilities (Chapter 2), but also remain attentive to context outside that of the person. For example, a given type of conversation—small talk, interview, phone versus face-to-face—may either reveal or hide certain deficits or, more importantly, retained abilities (Chapters 4 and 10).

A theme running through the book is that wedded to meaningful interaction is respect—respect for dignity and personhood even in the face of decline. For many contributors, the focus has been on understanding and facilitating talk and interaction as important components of what it means to be human. For others, the focus is an awareness of how through the skillful use of talk and interaction, we might better care for persons with dementia and encourage a sense of autonomy, control, and dignity (Chapter 11). Each of us will have a different motivation, whether it be to talk with a loved one, provide care to a patient, or advance our understanding of talk under the conditions of dementia. Whatever one's individual concerns in reading this book maybe, I trust that we have shown the value that attentiveness to our interactions with those who have dementia can bring as we each strive to be even better conversation partners, to heighten our awareness of *their* concerns, and to embrace each of them as individuals.

Research Guidance and Resources

The work in this volume, like others, bridges the worlds of research, clinical practice, and personal care. In addition to offering interactional practices that may aid personal and professional conversations with persons with dementia, all chapters in Part II serve as examples of methods to use in future studies—whether discourse, conversation, or syntactic analysis; ethnography; or a combination of these. Moreover, Chapters 3 and 10 offer explicit guidance to novice researchers and clinicians.

I want to conclude by drawing attention to several resources that can assist future researchers as they strive to better understand dementia.

The Carolinas Conversation Collection

The Carolinas Conversation Collection (CCC), introduced in Chapter 3 and used in several of the studies within Part II, offers a wealth of interactional audio and video data. The importance of this site is that the data have been approved for secondary research. The data provide for

> short-term and long-term research objectives, for specialists in communications disorders and gerontology, information technology, medical and health care researchers from multiple professions, linguists, psychologists, and archivists. Currently (Fall 2011), the Collection includes more than 200 conversational interviews with older persons having any of 12 chronic diseases, and more than 400 conversational interviews with older persons having cognitive impairment. (https://carolinaconversations.musc.edu/about/collection)

The interactional data housed within the CCC provides the researcher a wealth of naturally occurring, spoken data from older persons from a range of racial, ethnic, and linguistic groups that are otherwise often unavailable. Pope's and Davis' collection (2011) demonstrates the immeasurable value of collecting data that is protected for secondary research purposes—a practice we hope becomes more widespread.

The Portal of Geriatrics Online Education (POGOe)

The Portal of Geriatrics Online Education (POGOe) is an online database that aids geriatric educators (https://www.pogoe.org/). It contains more than 950 geriatrics educational materials that faculty across U.S. medical schools and the Centers for Geriatric Nursing Excellence have compiled. These materials include various instructional and assessment tools, including virtual and standardized patients, games, tutorials, case-based teaching, self-directed learning, and traditional lectures (Ramaswamy et al., 2015).

Dementia Research Networks

The creation of dementia registries as a means to compare case studies on prognoses, care, and research are also facilitating collaboration. For example, the National Institute of Health Research, the largest funder of health and care research in the U.K., established the Dementia and Neurodegenerative Research Network (DeNDRoN) which "aims to improve the speed, quality, and integration of research in dementias and other neurodegenerative diseases, resulting in improvements in prevention, diagnosis, treatment and care for patients" (Iliffe et al., 2011, p. 2). DeNDRoN primarily contains research from clinical trials, but it is open to including other well-designed studies. Such databases could connect the experimental and interactional research communities and encourage collaborative projects.

References

Iliffe, S., Curry, L., Kharicha, K., Rait, G., Wilcock, J., Lowery, D., … Ritchie, C. (2011). Developing a dementia research registry: A descriptive case study from North Thames DeNDRoN and the EVIDEM programme. *BMC Medical Research Methodology, 11*(9). https://doi.org/10.1186/1471-2288-11-9.

Pope, C., & Davis, B. H. (2011). Finding a balance: The Carolinas conversation collection. *Corpus Linguistics and Linguistic Theory, 7*(1), 143–161.

Ramaswamy, R., Leipzig, R. M., Howe, C. L., Sauvigne, K., Usiak, C., & Soriano, R. P. (2015). The portal of geriatrics online education: A 21st-century resource for teaching geriatrics. *Journal of the American Geriatrics Society, 63*(2), 335–340.

Glossary

Affiliation According with the demonstrated stance of the speaker of a prior turn

Agrammatism Speech containing mainly content words (e.g., nouns, verbs) with a lack of function words (e.g., prepositions, conjunctions, articles)

Alignment According with the expressed next sequential turn, for example, following a question with an answer

Assessment An evaluative utterance (e.g., "*That is a beautiful painting.*")

Authoritative knowledge Information received from people, books, a supreme being, or such sources. The strength of its value depends on cultural and/or contextual evaluation of the source

Change-of-state token Vocalizations designed to display a move to a new or different subjective state as a communicative action within talk (e.g., *oh*, *ouch*)

Content boundedness Talk that is contained, defined, circumscribed within the characteristics (e.g., topic, turn design) of the conversation

Conversation analysis Analysis of interaction that pays particular attention to the words, body movement, gaze, and gesture in consideration of where these resources are employed within the sequential position in the interaction (see Chapter 1, Methodological Approaches)

Discourse analysis As applied in Chapter 5, an analysis of language at levels smaller than the sentence. Analysts look to bits of language, such as lexical choices (words), order of words (grammar), sounds (phonetics and

T. Stickle (ed.), *Learning from the Talk of Persons with Dementia*,
The Language of Mental Health, https://doi.org/10.1007/978-3-030-43977-4

phonology), parts of words (morphology), and the meanings of expressions (semantics) in order to see how these elements both flow together and across participants to create meaning (see Chapter 1, Methodological Approaches)

Discourse ecology Language use (speech or written) designed to create knowledge niches and, consequently, perceptual atmospheres of a particular topic

Discourse markers Words or phrases that signal the relationship between the speaker's message and the rest of the communication. They help the listener connect the current utterance to the rest of the discourse (e.g., *well, I mean*). (See also "pragmatic markers".)

Epistemics (epistemic status/epistemic authority/ of social interaction) Words, expressions, phrases that express speakers' subjective assessments of the strength or reliability of certainty regarding the truth value of the information in their propositions

Ethnography Illumination of social life and culture in a particular social system based on multiple detailed observations (see Chapter 1, Methodological Approaches)

First pair part A turn that initiates an action

Go-aheads A two-syllable phrase used to encourage a conversation partner to carry on with the talk (e.g., *uh-huh, mmm-hmm, oh really*)

Grand tour Questions that provide the structure for responses that are in-depth, descriptive sequences that explain such things as a series of events, description of a group of people, telling how one is experiencing an event or condition

Informed consent The process by which a patient/research subject learns about and understands the purpose, benefits, and potential risks of participating in a research protocol and provides assent or agreement to be part of that research

Institutionalization The state of being placed or kept in a residential institution

Interactional sociolinguistics An approach to the study of discourse which analyses power within linguistic practices

Interlocutor Another name for a co-participant in conversation; one with whom another converses

Intersubjectivity Coordinating or adapting one's subjectivity with other's subjectivity within interaction

Joint attention The shared focus of two or more individuals on an object, topic, affective event. It is achieved when individuals alert one another to the focal object by means of eye-gazing, pointing, or other verbal or nonverbal indications

Lexicon One's mental collection of words

Minimal response A turn composed of vocal material which indicates little beyond acknowledgment of the prior turn (e.g. *uh-huh, yeah*)

Neurocognitive disorders A group of disorders in which the brain fundamentally changes due to any singular etiology or combination of etiologies. In turn, particular behaviors and emotional responses are affected

Palilalia A speech disorder characterized by involuntary repetition of one's own words, phrases, or sentences

Personal agency One's capability to originate and direct actions for given purposes

Practical accomplishments The ways in which objects are oriented to and shaped by participants through interaction

Pragmatics The study of language concerned with the cultural expectations that guide what is appropriate to say to whom

Pragmatic markers Pragmatic markers are linguistic clues which signal the speaker's probable communicative intentions (e.g., *I regret, I admit, incidentally*). (See also "discourse markers".)

Quilting A particular word or phrase used often by a person to elicit talk from a co-participant (e.g., *How about those apples?, Are you living the dream?*)

Recipient design The process by which speakers structure their talk in a way that is sensitive to the particular others involved in the social encounter

Reformulations A change in an utterance mid talk by the speaker (see also "repair")

Repair A correction completed by self or other within an interaction and used to fix an error or to clarify a misunderstanding. This refers to the set of practices whereby interlocutors attend to possible trouble in speaking, hearing, or understanding in conversation

Repairables Areas of trouble resulting from cognitive impairment

Repeats A second saying of a previous utterance

Restarts The practice of speakers to produce a fragment prior to a complete utterance

Second pair part A responding utterance

Semantics The branch of linguistics and logic concerned with meaning

Situated resources The ways in which objects are used by participants in interaction

Somatic unit Units in residential centers that focus on the connection of mind and body for holistic care

Tag questions A question converted from a statement by an appended interrogative formula (e.g., *It's nice out, isn't it?*)

Transitivity The property of a verb that relates to the number and types of objects it requires (e.g., *laugh* requires no objects: He laughed; *eat* requires one object: I ate my lunch; *give* requires two objects: a direct object and indirect object: I give my dog //a treat)

Turn construction unit A component of a speaker's turn after which the turn may be construed as complete

Wayfinding Events in conversation in which speakers have become lost in their own story or cannot immediately retrieve the gist of the conversation or the schema of a familiar event but do find their way back to that thread of talk

Wh-question A question in English introduced by a wh-word and requiring more information in reply than simply yes or no

Wordfinding difficulties A cover term used to signal a range of disfluencies including substitutions of incorrect or inappropriate words, or the inability to produce the desired word to adequately express a thought

Index

T. Stickle (ed.), *Learning from the Talk of Persons with Dementia*,
The Language of Mental Health, https://doi.org/10.1007/978-3-030-43977-4

The manufacturer's authorised representative in the EU is Springer Nature Customer Service Centre GmbH, Europaplatz 3, 69115 Heidelberg, Germany. If you have any concerns regarding our products, please contact ProductSafety@springernature.com

Printed and bound by CPI Group (UK) Ltd, Croydon, CR0 4YY
30/09/2026
02225459-0005